Supporting Women to Give Birth at Home

Supporting Women to Give Birth at Home describes and discusses the main challenges and issues that midwives and maternity services encounter when preparing for and attending a homebirth. To ensure that a homebirth is a real option for women, midwives need to be able to believe in a woman's ability to give birth at home and to promote this birth option, providing evidence-based information about benefits and risks.

This practical guide will help midwives to have the necessary skills, resources and confidence to support homebirth. The book includes:

- the present birth choices a woman has
- the implications homebirth has upon midwifery practice
- how midwives can prepare and support women and their families
- the midwife's role and responsibilities
- national and local policies, guidelines and available resources
- pain management options.

With a range of recent homebirth case studies brought together in the final chapter, this accessible text provides a valuable insight into those considering homebirth. *Supporting Women to Give Birth at Home* will be of interest to students studying issues around normal birth and will be an important resource for clinically based midwives, in particular community-based midwives, homebirth midwifery teams, independent midwives and all who are interested in homebirth as a genuine choice.

Mary Steen is Professor of Midwifery at the Faculty of Health and Social Care at the University of Chester, UK. She has practised as a midwife for 23 years and worked in a community setting since 1994, attending numerous homebirths. She has recently helped to develop a successful community-based health and well-being programme intended to increase the numbers of active births and homebirths.

Supporting Women to Give Birth at Home

A practical guide for midwives

Edited by Mary Steen

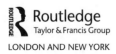

Routledge
Taylor & Francis Group

LONDON AND NEW YORK

First published 2012
by Routledge
2 Park Square, Milton Park, Abingdon, Oxon OX14 4RN

Simultaneously published in the USA and Canada
by Routledge
711 Third Avenue, New York, NY 10017

Routledge is an imprint of the Taylor & Francis Group, an informa business

British Library Cataloguing in Publication Data
A catalogue record for this book is available from the British Library

Library of Congress Cataloging in Publication Data
Supporting women to give birth at home : a practical guide for midwives / edited by Mary Steen.
  p. ; cm.
Includes bibliographical references.
1. Childbirth at home. 2. Midwifery. I. Steen, Mary.
[DNLM: 1. Home Childbirth. 2. Delivery, Obstetric—methods. 3. Midwifery—methods. 4. Women—psychology. WQ 155]
RG661.5.S87 2012
618.2–dc23
2011018287

ISBN: 978–0–415–56029–0 (hbk)
ISBN: 978–0–415–56030–6 (pbk)
ISBN: 978–0–203–32403–5 (ebk)

Typeset in Sabon by Prepress Projects Ltd, Perth, UK

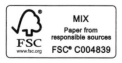

Printed and bound in Great Britain by
TJ International Ltd, Padstow, Cornwall

Contents

4 Supporting homebirth   81
Mary Steen and Kath Jones

Illustrations

Tables

Contributors

Kim Gibbon (MA Counselling Studies with distinction, Dip HE with distinction, PGDip Ed, PGCert Clinical Governance with distinction, RM, RGN) has worked for 33 years in the clinical arena in nursing and midwifery with a period of specialisation in fetal medicine. This depth of clinical experience is complemented by extensive management experience as a Senior Manager, Head of Midwifery, as well as practising as a qualified counsellor. Now a Senior Lecturer in Midwifery, she continues to work as a Supervisor of Midwives and NMC Fitness to Practise panellist.

Jane Harris (MSc, PGCert Ed, ADM, RM, RGN) is Deputy Head of Midwifery and Reproductive Health and Programme Leader for BSc (Hons) Midwifery at the University of Chester. She has worked in midwifery education for 20 years and prior to that was a midwifery ward manager. Jane has recently commenced her PhD studies and the subject area will be the experiences of bereaved fathers following a stillbirth and neonatal death up to 28 days.

Kath Jones MBE has been a midwife for 35 years and is currently employed by the Maternity Services, Wrexham Maelor Hospital, Betsi Cadwaladr University Health Board, North Wales.

Brigid McKeown (BSc (Hons), PG Dip (Health and Social Care Management), RM, RN) practised as a community midwife for over 20 years. She is currently the Lead Midwife for Community Midwifery and Public Health and Supervisor of Midwives for the Northern Health and Social Care Trust, Northern Ireland. A Supervisor of Midwives for almost 10 years, she was involved in the development of the regional supervisors of midwives' Annual Review Record and participates in the local auditing of supervisory standards. In her most recent management role she has been involved in guideline development within the Northern Health and Social Care Trust.

Julia Magill-Cuerden (FRCM, NTF, PhD, MA, DN, Dip Ed, MTD, RM, RN) is an Emeritus Scholar of the University of West London. Formerly she was a Principal Lecturer in midwifery and Senior Research Fellow in education at Thames Valley University. She has been a Supervisor of Midwives and has held strong links in clinical practice through the roles of supervision and link lecturer. She has worked in the community.

Mary Steen is Professor of Midwifery at the Faculty of Health and Social Care at the University of Chester. She has practised as a midwife for 23 years and has worked in a community setting since 1994, attending numerous homebirths. She has recently helped to develop a successful community-based health and well-being programme intended to increase the numbers of active births and homebirths.

Verena Wallace (MSc (Health Policy, Planning & Finance), MSc (Advanced Midwifery Practice), ADM, RM, RN) has worked as a midwife in Scotland, England and Northern Ireland. While a community midwife in London she was seconded to national policy implementation projects (CESDI and Changing Childbirth) and in Leeds practised as a consultant midwife in public health and then as deputy chief nurse for women's services. Prior to her appointment as local supervising authority midwifery officer, Verena was a head of midwifery in Northern Ireland with over 10 years' experience as a supervisor of midwives.

Foreword

Books on homebirth always generate interest because, despite very good evidence supporting homebirth safety, it remains a controversial topic. Over the past couple of years, newspaper headlines have been made by studies purporting to question homebirth's safety for babies. Positive headlines about the safety of homebirth do not make it into the papers.

In the UK, the homebirth choice is a cherished component of midwifery services and has a very long history of being a choice for women regarding their preferred place of birth. Despite this, the numbers of women choosing it remain very low, though rates vary enormously across the country. Within the UK, homebirth rates have never recovered from the blow dealt them by the Peel Report in 1970, which encouraged women to birth in hospital.

Different patterns of homebirth provision exist across the developed world, with the Netherlands leading the way in having about 25 per cent of all women birthing at home. But, like the UK, most western countries have seen a centralisation of birthing in large maternity hospitals.

It is, therefore, very timely that this edited book on a variety of aspects of homebirth is published. I could think of no better editor to undertake this task than Dr Mary Steen. With her roots in domiciliary and homebirth practice, she speaks from personal experience. But it is her work in public health, especially around families and adaptation to parenthood, that makes her contribution here unique. She views homebirth through a social model lens and then is transparent in her own chapters and in her editing.

You will find in this book a range of chapters covering important aspects of homebirth provision, and it is therefore suitable for women and maternity care practitioners alike. Dr Steen has assembled experts in the field to write about their own passions regarding homebirth – all of which show through in the lucid and attention-holding writing.

I would recommend every midwife, midwifery student and women unde-cided about place of birth for their baby to read this book. It will reacquaint you with the specialness of birthing in your own environment, and will remind midwives of one of the most satisfying aspects of their professional work.

Dr Denis Walsh
Associate Professor in Midwifery
Nottingham University, UK

Preface

Home as a 'place of birth' is a topical area of interest both nationally and internationally. There is an on-going homebirth debate with regards to risks and benefits for the mother and child, and Mary Nolan has recently stated that:

> The debate is about choice; it is about women's freedoms and midwifery autonomy and in order to be fully informed, it needs midwives' voices to be heard.
>
> (Nolan, 2011, p. 6)

Nolan challenges individual midwives and the midwifery profession on not participating in, let alone directing, the homebirth debate. The contributors of this book are experienced midwives who have attended and supported many women to have a homebirth during their midwifery careers. This book gives these midwives an opportunity to be heard and their knowledge and views to be considered and debated.

Let us not forget that home is the natural place to give birth and at the end of pregnancy woman innately 'nest' and prepare for the forthcoming birth of their infant. However, in the twentieth century, the shift from home to hospital and the increasing medicalisation of childbirth has influenced how birth is viewed and experienced.

Ina May Gaskin (2008, p. 4) has stated:

> Living in a technological society we tend to think the best of everything is the most expensive kind available. This is generally true whether we are talking about cell phones, cameras, cars or computers. When it comes to birth it ain't necessarily so.

Davies (2004, p. 151) asks: 'We can take the midwife out of the hospital, but can we take the hospital out of the midwife?'

The contributors of this book believe that this can be achieved. The overall aim of this book is to discuss and describe the main statutory and practical challenges and issues that midwives and maternity services face when supporting women who request a homebirth, and then whilst facilitating a homebirth.

The security of being based in a consultant-led unit with on-call obstetric and paediatric back-up will be reassuring and familiar for many midwives, but an increasing number of midwives are unhappy with this approach, which often conflicts with the philosophy of normal birth and promotes a medical rather than a social model of care.

Midwives need to enable and empower women to give birth in their own homes. To do this they themselves need to believe in a woman's ability to give birth at home and promote this birth option. It is also essential that they have the necessary skills and confidence to support women who choose to have a homebirth. Midwifery education and maternity services may need to reflect on how they perceive and promote homebirth as a genuine choice for women who wish to give birth in their own home. One tangible benefit is that homebirth increases the possibility of continuity of care and carer, the effects of which have been shown to influence birth positively. The Royal College of Midwives in the UK is supporting the normality of birth and running a 'Campaign for Normal Birth' which promotes homebirth as a genuinely safe option for many women.

In the UK, homebirth rates remain relatively low, and a practical guide that assists midwives to support women will be a valuable resource to promote homebirths. It is envisaged that this book will help midwives gain knowledge based on the best available evidence and also provide an insight into some women's and midwives' experiences of homebirths. In addition, this book should increase midwives' confidence and ability to promote homebirth as an option. Increasing women's knowledge and awareness that their home is a safe place to give birth and ensuring that midwives have the necessary skills and resources to support homebirths may help steadily increase rates over the next decade or so.

This book is introduced by an exploration of the history of birth, the transition from the home environment to the hospital setting, the present birth choices a woman has and the implications of these for midwifery practice. This sets the scene for the book to then focus upon homebirth itself.

Further chapters cover how midwives can prepare and support women, their partners and families to have a homebirth. The midwife's role and responsibilities are explored, as well as how supervision can support midwives to prepare and attend homebirths. National and local policies, guidelines and available resources will be referred to. One chapter specifically focuses on pain management options and another chapter is dedicated to describing and discussing some women's homebirth experiences. These homebirths were planned and unplanned, demonstrating a range of possible outcomes and giving an insight into the individualised care needed for these women.

If women receive unbiased advice and information based on the best available evidence regarding homebirth, they are more likely to be satisfied with their care regardless of whether the birth takes place in their own home. Maternity services need to provide calm, caring, confident midwives who have the skills to attend homebirths and are supported by a good referral and transfer system to a consultant-led unit if the need should arise. This will ensure that homebirth is a genuine option for women and promote normal childbirth.

Reference

Davies, L. (2004) 'Allowed' shouldn't be allowed! *MIDIRS Midwifery Digest*, 14, 151–156.
Gaskin, I.M. (2008) *Ina May's Guide to Childbirth*. Vermilion: London.
Nolan, M.L. (2011) *Homebirth: The Politics of Difficult Choices*. Routledge: London.

Acknowledgements

A very special thank you to the women who agreed to share their birth stories and Andrea McLaughlin, Head of Midwifery and Reproductive Health Education, University of Chester, for her support and advice. I am very grateful to have had Matt Bornshin draw the illustrations included and the support and knowledge of midwives who have contributed to this book. Last but not least to have had excellent support from James Watson and Grace McInnes and the Routledge team.

Chapter 1   **History of homebirth**

Jane Harris

Introduction

This chapter outlines the origins of midwifery and describes how homebirth was the norm for millennia. It explores the impact that medicine has had on childbirth, particularly as it has grown in strength and influence over the past 400 years. Looking at more recent developments, the chapter notes the social, professional, political and technological pressures that moved birth into hospitals as well as the recent resurgence of interest in homebirth. By exploring how homebirth came to be considered 'dangerous', the chapter helps the reader to see that it is not, and to understand how it can be rehabilitated.

> In the home setting . . . the rhythms of a labouring woman's body are honoured and waited on, and where birth is non-interventionist and centred on people, instead of mechanical processes.
>
> Kitzinger (2002, p. 8)

In the beginning

Life has a tendency to run in cycles, and we are now witnessing a more natural approach to all aspects of life from birth to the environment. Traditionally, throughout history, birth has been a social event that takes place within the nurturing setting of the home, which was the centre of life and where everything happened (Chamberlain *et al.*, 1997). The event of birth was a communal celebration, a rite of passage (Van Gennep, 2004), with a predominantly female support mechanism (Donnison, 1988).

This approach worked fairly successfully for centuries in the main (Donnison, 1988). Mortality was high across the social and gender spectrum, with life expectancy in general being relatively low. Thus, high mortality rates in females were not only associated with childbirth (Gélis, 1991). Traditionally females have been the main carers in labour, with documentation of trained Hebrew midwives in the bible. In the Book of Genesis (King James Version, 35:16) it is stated that during the birthing process of Benjamin, the midwife told Rachel that she would have a son. This birth took place in or around 1800 BC and unfortunately Rachel did not survive. From a historical perspective the Bible is and remains a valuable source of recorded births and deaths including maternal mortality. Within Egyptian society midwifery was recognised as a female occupation of high standing, and this included attending and supporting the members of the royal households (Towler and Bramall, 1986). Documented scenes of Egyptian childbirth and midwifery support have been preserved in time from as early as 1900 BC (Gélis, 1991).

Midwives in Greece were held in high repute within the hierarchy of their early medical systems. Both the mother of Socrates and the wife of Pericles were midwives. The great scholar Aristotle spoke of the wisdom and intelligence of the midwives of Greece (College of Midwives, 2008). Within the system at that time midwives were categorised into two grades: those who were deemed to have a higher level of skill and knowledge, who were mainly responsible for women experiencing complicated labours, and those who assisted at normal births (Towler and Bramall, 1986). A parallel exists between practice in ancient times and the roles of midwives today in westernised societies, which has seen the increasing development of advanced midwifery practitioners who carry out instrumental deliveries and diagnose complications within the context of the hospital environment, working alongside midwives who remain the gatekeepers of normal birth (Walsh, 2007).

As medicine advanced within Greece during the next two centuries up to 300 BC, the demise of the midwife took place, much to the dismay of the women of Greece, who had strong objections to male attendants. It is apparent that as soon as medics take an interest in childbirth, they have great difficulty in working alongside the original practitioners of this art, the midwives. In response, one woman, Agnodice, disguised herself as a man in order to train under a famous physician and anatomist named Hierophilus. She did, however, reveal her true identity to the women she assisted and eventually she was denounced by the medical profession and was charged, although the mothers of Athens called for clemency. As a result, it was ruled that 'three of the sex should practise this art in Athens' (Potter, 1764). The voice of the client has always been a powerful force within the history of childbirth and in particular homebirth (Kitzinger, 2008).

Midwives have even been immortalised as gods in both Greek and Roman lore. Artemis was a goddess associated with childbirth, as was Hera the wife of Zeus. Hera was also recognised in Roman mythology under her Roman name of Juno Lucina. She was the symbol of the Roman matron, and women would call out to her in labour 'Juno Lucina, ser opem' (help assist the labour) (Towler and Bramall, 1986). The symbol on the hat badge of midwives in the UK is Juno Lucina holding a baby. This represents an educated and skilled woman from a culture and time when a midwife was a symbol of status within that society (McMaster, 1912).

Symbolism plays a major role in history and its interpretation, as does the status of women. It is clear that throughout history women have been encouraged to be educated and resourceful only when it is deemed necessary by the strong patriarchal force that has always been dominant and embedded within the majority of societies around the world (Pilley Edwards, 2005). The development of capitalism, industrialisation and professionalism led to greater benefits for men than for women. This then ensured that policy-making was led by men and therefore the needs of women became secondary. It is in this context that the history of birth, and in particular homebirth, has developed (Pilley Edwards, 2005). What has become obvious over time is that the picture of childbirth greatly altered as soon as medicine decided to create a specialised role within this previously female dominated forum (Donnison, 1988). Yet again this links closely with the long history of men controlling women.

The changing face of birth

The stronghold of the home environment for birth was perpetuated throughout the Middle Ages, medieval times, the Renaissance, through to the early eighteenth century, even though hospitals became established institutions during this time. Their first incarnation was as a place where the poor were cared for, along with the dying and people who had suffered accidents, and this had connotations of death. Birth was perceived as a natural element of life and was not categorised as an illness requiring hospital treatment (Towler and Bramall, 1986).

The medical profession was developing and growing in strength, particularly within the specialist fields of surgery and medicine. Because of this growth, midwives were left alone to carry on with their work in the domain of childbirth. It is a incorrect to suggest that all midwives were uneducated and unskilled in their field. Even the traditional midwives were given training via the apprentice approach, whereby family members would pass down the skills and their teachings mainly based upon their experiences (Gélis, 1991). The majority of midwives gave the women the best possible care for that time in history (Gélis, 1991).

The more educated women who practised midwifery wanted to ensure that the role of the midwife developed and that the teaching of the skills and diagnostics was made more formal so that midwives could be monitored and regulated. Jane Sharp was the first English midwife to write a textbook on midwifery, in 1671. It was titled *The Midwives Book or the Whole Art of Midwifery Discovered* (Sharp, 1671). The purpose of the book was to instruct midwives to ensure that women were cared for by skilled attendants, which was in sharp contrast to the image of midwives during this period (Bosanquet, 2009). She strongly believed that a woman should be given individualised care and recommended mobilisation with the woman taking up the positions that her body dictated; this was in contrast to the views of male authors of the time, who prescribed that only certain positions be used for birth. The issues of advocacy, accountability and partnerships in care were documented and championed by Sharp. Also included in the book was a series of drawings showing fetal positions, advice about all stages of labour and the importance of nutrition and hydration during labour.

The Church played a major role in demonising midwives and the services that they had to offer the communities in which they lived. This stemmed from man's intrigue with birth and its links to procreation. The Church became judicial in relation to governing the practices of midwifery, stating that women who could become a midwife must 'be of good character' (Towler and Bramall, 1986) This premise has been carried on to the present day as in order to register as a midwife the lead for midwifery education must sign a declaration of good character for each student at the end of the programme of education (Nursing and Midwifery Council, 2009).

Medicine's fascination with birth really came into play during the eighteenth century, which saw the emergence of the man-midwife, an early incarnation of the obstetrician. The Chamberlain brothers devised a set of forceps for assisting difficult births within the home environment, and William Smellie attended several homebirths and commented on the use of birthing stools and the left lateral position when using the bed. He concurred that both positions were very helpful in assisting women through the process of birth (Towler and Bramall, 1986). Middle- and upper-class women were willing to pay for the services of the new man-midwife because they perceived a trained male as superior to a midwife. This view is reflective of the status of women during these times, predominantly uneducated in a formal sense with no voting rights and no real social rights (Towler and Bramall, 1986). The historian Don Shelton's recent revelation (Shelton, 2010) about the pregnant women used as models for the anatomical atlases produced by William Smellie and William Hunter is enlightening. He posits that these women were procured through the practice of 'burking', that is, soliciting the murder of people for medical investigation. This highlights yet again the fact that women and their bodies were perceived as vessels for unlawful and unethical experimentation and professional gain by some medical men, such as William Smellie.

Whilst Smellie was assisting in and writing about homebirths, maternity hospitals were being opened in western Europe. They were mainly established by philanthropists who deemed that the poor and lower classes did not live in the right conditions for home deliveries and consequently they established lying-in hospitals. This act was mainly for charitable and social reasons rather than being based on medical evidence. From 1739 to 1765 four of these institutions were established in London. Only one of the original lying-in hospitals remains open today, and that is Queen Charlotte's Hospital for Women. This type of hospital was also being established in Dublin (the Rotunda Maternity Hospital) and in Edinburgh (Towler and Bramall, 1986). Some of these establishments provided short training periods for female pupils. They were trained and examined by doctors, and this continued until the twentieth century (Cowell and Wainwright, 1981). It would seem that a body of women who were trained and deemed competent practitioners were believed to be unable to govern their profession in an accountable way. The picture that is usually presented of midwives at this time is of a motley crew of uneducated, unclean and drunken women from the poorest backgrounds, but this was not the case. Many of the midwives had received a formal education and had then undertaken training to become a midwife. The care they provided was of a standard that was appropriate at that period in time (Donnison, 1988). The influence of medicine was already having an impact on the development of midwifery and the power battle between midwives and the developing specialty that was to become obstetrics had begun. These developments had a growing impact upon midwives practising their art as they struggled to compete with their male counterparts. They persevered and, by the end of the eighteenth century, midwifery had survived (Donnison, 1988).

Maternity hospitals were not a new concept in Europe. Major cities in France and Germany had maternity hospitals that had been established since the middle of the sixteenth century; however, they were not particularly popular with the women of the day. One of the most famous and earliest maternity hospitals was the Hotel Dieu in Paris. It was mainly a teaching establishment, where the poor of the city were gathered so that Ambroise Paré could train midwives (Towler and Bramall, 1986).

In the nineteenth century, 15 additional maternity hospitals were established in the UK, mainly in the highly populated cities. The majority of women, 99 per cent of whom had uncomplicated pregnancies, were still giving birth at home (Campbell and Macfarlane, 1995), which was safer because rates of puerperal sepsis leading to maternal mortality were increasing in the maternity hospitals (Towler and Bramall, 1986). Infection was transferred from patient to patient via the unwashed hands of the carers, in particular by doctors, who not uncommonly carried out postmortem examinations and then performed internal examinations upon the women without washing their hands. The answer was simple – increase the levels of hygiene, which meant hand washing between patients and procedures. This simple task reduced the incidence of infection and is still the main bulwark against cross-infection today (Johnson and Taylor, 2010).

The medical culture of birth

During the nineteenth century major developments took place within the realm of maternity care. They were the use of chloroform for the relief of pain in labour, as used by Queen Victoria, and the increasing success of caesarean sections as life-saving operations. These developments were costly and were carried out in the hospital environment, which meant that they had little impact upon domiciliary midwifery and poorer women (Towler and Bramall, 1986).

As the legislation and governing of medicine was developing, so too was the issue of the status of the midwife. Florence Nightingale supported the traditional premise of midwifery, but she also wanted to extend the role and raise the standard of practice by ensuring that the right kind of women entered the profession and that they were trained to give a high level of skilful care (Nightingale, 1871). From the late nineteenth century, many educated women practised as midwives and they wanted to ensure that the profession became self-governing with a legislative foundation. A small group of midwives led by Miss Zepherina Veitch and Rosalind Paget began the Midwives Institute and petitioned parliament to endorse and pass the Midwives Act. It was not an easy process and it took perseverance to finally get the Act through in 1902. The Act set up the Central Midwives Board, which was the governing body for all trained midwives. From this came the midwives' rules, which set out the standards and the parameters of practice. This was a major development for the profession but it was tainted by the dominance of the medical presence surrounding the changes (Cowell and Wainwright, 1981).

During the early part of the twentieth century, midwives were still self-employed and their income was dependent on what women could afford to pay for their services; furthermore, payment was not always in a monetary form. Also during this period antenatal care and the precursor of antenatal education were introduced in Scotland. The benefits of this care were disseminated and the programme was rolled out across the UK. Alongside these new developments in maternity care, the rate of maternal mortality was causing the growing number of obstetricians concern. From 1869 to 1900, the recorded maternal mortality rate was 5.5 per 1000 live births and the average infant mortality rate was 153 per 1000 live births. The reasons for high mortality rates were poverty, unsanitary living conditions, high fertility rates and poor nutrition leading to anaemia and rickets, which caused contraction to the pelvis, resulting in prolonged and sometimes obstructed labours (Tew, 1998). Unfortunately, these figures did not alter for the next 30 years (Holland, 1935). Searching for explanations for these statistics led many professionals to blame birth attendants for not acting wisely, the women for their behaviour and the birth environment (Tew, 1998). They felt that the solution would be to increase hospital births under the care of the obstetrician, which would give women greater access to pain relief and operative interventions (Tew, 1998). This approach did not reduce the poor housing and social conditions that a great many of the women would be returning to once their hospital stay was over. The health professional who remained constant in the lives of the majority of women continued to be the midwife working within the community setting.

Practices in the home setting were reliant on the process of normality and the woman wanting a natural approach to pain relief. Advances in antenatal care and labour were accompanied by the development of anaesthesia and the use of opiates for pain relief. These options for pain relief were very firmly fixed within the hospital domain so, for women who wanted to choose these methods of pain relief, hospital was the best option. Alongside these developments the education of midwives was increasingly influenced by the medicalisation of birth. Midwives were taught to carry out procedures such as episiotomy, but not all midwives were taught to suture said episiotomies, which meant that a doctor had to be called (Tew, 1998). There was one guiding light during this period, an obstetrician called Dr Grantley Dick-Read, who believed that women laboured in a more positive way if they had support and were talked through the contractions (Dick-Read, 1964). This reinforced the homebirth approach, as women choosing this approach were assured of one-to-one care and support (Central Midwives Board, 1962).

Over the next few decades maternal and perinatal mortality did decrease to a small fraction of what it had been 50 years previously, but this is not entirely attributable to the medicalisation of childbirth, as we have been seduced into believing (Tew, 1998). During this time social welfare also improved, and improvements in housing conditions, education and employment all had a positive impact upon mortality rates, as did improved maternal nutrition, there having always been a positive correlation between maternal nutrition and maternal and perinatal outcome (Tew, 1998). In this period homebirth in uncomplicated cases was as safe as delivery in the new hospitals (Campbell and Macfarlane, 1994). Resource-wise it was more economical to provide a domiciliary service than to have all women delivering in hospital; however, from 1927 to 1946, hospital birth rates as a proportion of all births continued to increase, from 15 to 54 per cent (Peretz, 1990).

The governance and legislation of midwifery continued to develop, in order to ensure that the general public was receiving safe and effective care from midwives. This was achieved by supervision and a national education curriculum for all midwives in training. The training was extended to one year for qualified nurses and two years for non-nurses. Midwives were now employed and paid a wage, which was a major improvement for their lifestyle. This also meant that all women had access to a trained midwife for their delivery within the community (Central Midwives Board, 1962). In spite of the developments within the profession, the obstetric discourse was starting to impact and erode the role of the midwife, who as a result became more of a handmaiden to the obstetric team rather than the lead professional (Robinson, 1990).

During this developmental period, aspects of care were improved such as extended antenatal care and postnatal care up to 28 days. The training of midwives was scrutinised on a regular basis by the Central Midwives Board (CMB), and this led to the training being split into two parts to cover both normal aspects of care and complications that may arise. The trainees had to undertake examinations in both clinical and theoretical elements of practice. Part 2 of the year was predominantly domiciliary care to ensure that midwives were skilled and competent to care for women in the home environment (Central Midwives Board, 1962).

Domiciliary care leading up to the 1960s was carried out by trained and experienced midwives who felt very comfortable in supporting women to give birth in their homes. They were also trained to recognise complications and to refer the women to a medical practitioner, which also reduced mortality rates (Central Midwives Board, 1962). The Cranbrook Report, published in 1959 (Cranbrook, 1959), recommended a hospital delivery rate of 70 per cent. During this time the percentage of homebirths was decreasing and, over a 70-year span from 1900 to 1970, the homebirth rate fell from 99 per cent to 12.4 per cent (Campbell and Macfarlane, 1994). The NHS continued to develop and went through many restructures, which impacted upon the way that the domiciliary midwifery services were funded. Along with a falling birth rate, this resulted in a shrinking service, with more midwives being employed within hospitals rather than in the community (Campbell and Macfarlane, 1994). By the late 1960s the hospital birth rate had risen to 85 per cent. In 1970, the Peel Report (Department of Health, 1970) recommended 100 per cent hospital delivery because of the supposed greater level of safety for both mother and child. This was the final measure that resulted in a 99 per cent hospital delivery rate and a 1 per cent home delivery rate throughout the next three decades.

The culture of birth up to the twentieth century in the UK, the rest of Europe and the USA had been homebirth. The main shift to hospital births occurred with the growth of obstetrics, improvements in healthcare and more maternity beds being made available for women throughout the western world (Tew, 1998). The only country to retain its tradition of homebirth and midwifery-led care was The Netherlands. Other factors also helped to promote this phenomenon, such as urbanisation: the younger generation were moving away from their country lives and their families to find employment in the industrialised towns. They no longer had their family support and were living in much smaller accommodation, which did not always lend itself to homebirths (Towler and Bramall, 1986). The two world wars also had an impact upon society, in particular the Second World War. The generation born after the war became known as the baby boomers and they wanted better conditions and easier access to treatment when complications developed (Towler and Bramall, 1986).

The most profound impact on homebirths came from the initiation of the UK's National Health Service (NHS) in 1947 (Donnison, 1988). This altered the way in which medicine was financed, allowing women to have greater access to all types of care. Doctors would now be employed or commissioned by the health service, which meant that predominantly obstetric work would take place within hospitals. Society began to associate hospitals with science, new developments and a return to health, rather than with death. Family size was also reducing quite dramatically, with more women using barrier methods of contraception (Oakley, 1986). In addition, women wanted a safe outcome to their pregnancies and they started to associate this with hospitals, advances in medicine and access to doctors (Pilley Edwards, 2005). Women were also becoming more educated about pain relief in labour and quickly realised that they were able to access more options within the hospital. Unlike the hospitals of the nineteenth century, which were aimed at the poorer classes, twentieth-century hospitals began to attract middle-class women (Towler and Bramall, 1986).

The technocratic approach to birth

This new era of maternity care saw the demise of homebirth along with the growing patriarchal control of midwives. During the 1970s and 1980s, midwifery and normal birth were railroaded by the growing use of biomedicine, the power of obstetrics within the hierarchy of the health service and the supported disbelief in the capacity of the female body to cope and manage birth without intervention (Oakley, 1986).

In the past, women had supported women to believe in themselves and their bodily cues during labour and birth. Now they were being told that their bodies could not cope and they needed to be strapped to machines and receive medication to control their contractions (Oakley, 1986). This approach was very mechanical, utilising the metaphor of the woman's body as a machine and the doctor in the role of engineer/mechanic; this was further perpetuated by the analogy of a factory process relating childbirth to a production line (Martin, 2001). The increasing use of technology made it increasingly difficult to continue with a homebirth as the technocratic approach was predominantly hospital bound. Over the next few years, birth within the home environment became not encouraged. Women who requested a homebirth were perceived as thoughtless with no conception of the dangers that they could be inflicting upon their unborn child and themselves (Pilley Edwards, 2005). This medical approach was influencing not only women but also the midwives who were caring for the women. This team approach to medicalisation became a powerful force, which women found to be impenetrable (Wesson, 2006).

Women's voices continued to debate the safety of delivering at home during the dominating years of hospital birth. Consumer groups such as the National Childbirth Trust, Maternity Alliance and Improvements for Maternity Services kept the issue alive through their members and the increasing interest of midwives who wanted to practise using their whole range of competencies (Oakley, 1986). This battle was further supported by the evidence that emerged from Marjorie Tew's study on statistics for place of birth. Before this study was carried out by Tew, an independent medical research statistician, the statistics that had been presented gave the view that hospital births were the safest option and had been the main reason for the reduction maternal and perinatal mortality. Tew's work broke through the resistance and revealed the false use of statistics to support a system that, at times, was in fact harming those it was supposed to benefit (Tew, 1998); this was further supported by Inch (1991). The medical journals kept resisting the information and eventually the only way for Tew publicise her results was to write a book.

From this point on, a great debate emerged. The subject matter is the definition of normal birth, as only from this understanding can come the definition of what is abnormal. This grey area leads to the distinction between a medical model of care, which is that pregnancy and birth can be considered normal only after the event, and a midwifery social model of care, that is, pregnancy and birth are normal until stated otherwise (Bryar, 1995). It makes it difficult to express a uniform definition of normal pregnancy and birth owing to the large variation in the women who have a healthy experience of childbirth (Pilley Edwards, 2005). Midwives need to own their authoritative knowledge and believe in their expertise of the normal childbirth continuum in whatever setting the woman has chosen (Jordan, 1997). This is also supplemented by their skills in identifying complications and dealing with emergency situations (Lavender and Chapple, 2008).

This then lends itself to the model of care that has been expounded in all the government reports that have emerged since, from *Changing Childbirth* (Department of Health, 1993) through to the *National Service Frameworks* (Department of Health, 2004) and *Maternity Matters* (Department of Health, 2007). All these advocate individualised care, viable options for place of birth and an equal partnership in the planning and pattern of care provided and agreed upon. This philosophy also relies on paternalism relinquishing its stronghold on the approaches to care. Paternalistic attitudes are not just fostered within obstetrics but are also evident within the profession of midwifery.

If all women are to be offered options that are based on evidence, then they must be allowed to process the information and make up their own minds about the type of care that is right for themselves and their circumstances. Midwives must also ensure that the environment in which these discussions take place is conducive and encouraging, not negative and persuasive (Pilley Edwards, 2005).

Slowly, over the last decade, homebirths have become more popular with the general public. This has come about by the growing involvement of consumers in the discussions and recommendations made in the pertinent government reports. Trusts have also realised the importance of quality-led consumer services and so consumer representation is mandatory on certain trust committees. This approach is also impacting upon professional health programmes of education including midwifery (Nursing and Midwifery Council, 2009). This is a positive approach which will ensure that the voices of the consumers of the service, women, are heard.

The perception paradigm is slowly beginning to shift, not only among women themselves, but also among midwives and some obstetricians, such that women who want to deliver at home are no longer viewed as zealots who want to break away from the safety of medicalised birth, but are acknowledged as having made an educated decision about their needs and the birth experience that they want rather than having such decisions thrust upon them (Lavender and Chapple, 2008).

The rate of homebirths is now slowly beginning to increase. The overall rate in the UK is now 2.5 per cent, although it varies around the country, ranging from 0.3 per cent in Renfrewshire in Scotland to 10.7 per cent in Powys, Wales. This is an overall rise of 9.7 per cent over a 12-month period. It is gratifying to see this increase, which indicates that women are receiving the choice that they have been asking for (Birth Choice UK, 2008). However, it is evident from lay websites that even now many women are not receiving balanced information and are therefore unable to make an informed choice about where to have their babies (Birth Choice UK, 2008). Midwives must resist the urge to overtly or covertly influence the decision-making of their clients in relation to place of birth (Lavender and Chapple, 2008). Their role is to inform and support women during this vulnerable time in their lives.

Conclusion

This chapter has presented the history of birth from early Egyptian and Greek times up to the current practices. It has shown how there is a rich narrative of positive homebirthing experiences, which were the norm until the twentieth century. It has explored the influence that medicine and developing technology has had on childbirth, along with the social, political and professional factors that have influenced the place of birth over the ages, some of which have promoted the whole concept of homebirth as a dangerous experience. In addition to these elements, the chapter has highlighted that homebirth can be a safe option.

References

Birth Choice (2008) *Big Rise in UK Births* (www.BirthChoiceUK.com; accessed 4 January 2011).

Bosanquet, A. (2009) Inspirations from the past. 1. Jane Sharp. *Practising Midwife*, 12(8), 33–5.

Bryar, R.M. (1995) *Theory for Midwifery Practice*. London: Macmillan Press.

Campbell, R. and Macfarlane, A. (1994) *Where to Be Born: The Debate and the Evidence*, 2nd edn. Oxford: National Perinatal Epidemiology Unit.

Central Midwives Board (1962) *Handbook Incorporating The Rules of the Central Midwives Board*. London: William Clowes & Sons.

Chamberlain, G. Wraight, A. and Crowley, P. (eds.) (1997) *Homebirths: The Report of the 1994 Confidential Enquiry by the National Birth Trust Fund*. London: Parthenon Publishing Group.

College of Midwives (2008) *Midwives of Great Antiquity and Historical Influence* (www.collegeofmidwives.org/legal_legislative01HxMfryIndex01/antiqmdw.htm; accessed 17 September 2010).

Cowell, B. and Wainwright, D. (1981) *Behind the Blue Door: History of the Royal College of Midwives, 1881–1981*. London: Baillière Tindall.

Cranbrook, Lord (Chair) (1959) *Report of the Maternity Services Committee*. London: HMSO.

Department of Health (1970) *Peel Report*. London: Department of Health.

Department of Health (1993) *Changing Childbirth: Report of the Expert Maternity Group, Vol. I*. London: HMSO.

Department of Health (2004) *National Services Framework for Children, Young People and Maternity Services*. London: Department of Health.

Department of Health (2007) *Maternity Matters: Choice, Access and Continuity of Care in a Safe Service*. London: Department of Health.

Dick-Read, G. (1964) *Childbirth without Fear*. London: William Heinemann Medical Books.

Donnison, J. (1988) *Midwives and Medicine Men: A History of the Struggle for the Control of Childbirth*, 2nd edn. New Barnett, UK: Historical Publications.

Gélis, J. (1991) *History of Childbirth: Fertility, Pregnancy and Birth in Early Modern Europe*. Cambridge: Polity Press.

Holland, E. (1935) Maternal mortality. *The Lancet*, 27 April, 973–6.

Inch, S. (1991) *Birthrights: A Parents Guide to Modern Childbirth*, 2nd edn. New York: Pantheon.

Johnson, R. and Taylor, W. (2010) *Skills for Midwifery Practice*, 3rd edn. London: Elsevier Churchill Livingstone.

Jordan, B. (1997) Authoritative knowledge and its construction. In Davis-Floyd, R. and Sargent, C.F. (eds.) *Childbirth and Authoritative Knowledge: Cross-Cultural Perspectives*. Berkeley, CA: University of California Press.

Kitzinger S. (2002) Why birth without hospital? In *Birth Your Way*. Dorling Kindersley: London, p. 8.

Kitzinger, S. (2008) Home birth: a social process, not a medical crisis. In Wickman, S. (ed.) *Midwifery Best Practice, Vol. 5* (e-book). London: Elsevier Health.

Lavender, T. and Chapple, J. (2008) How women choose where to give birth. In Wickman, S. (ed.) *Midwifery Best Practice, Vol. 5*. London: Butterworth Heinemann Elsevier.

McMaster, G.T. (1912) Ancient Greece. The first woman practitioner (Agnodice) of midwifery and the care of infants in Athens, 300 B.C. *American Medicine, New Series B*, 4, 202–5.

Martin, E. (2001) *The Woman in the Body: A Cultural Analysis of Reproduction*. Boston: Beacon Press.

Nightingale, F. (1871) *Introductory Notes on Lying-In Institutions*. London: Elibron Classics.

Nursing and Midwifery Council (NMC) (2009) *Standards for Pre-registration Midwifery Education*. London: NMC.

Oakley, A. (1986) *The Captured Womb: A History of the Medical Care of Pregnant Women*, 2nd edn. Oxford: Basil Blackwell.

Peretz, E. (1990) A maternity service for England and Wales: local authority maternity care in the inter-war period in Oxfordshire and Tottenham. In Garcia, J. Kilpatrick, R. and Richards, M. (eds.) *The Politics of Maternity Care: Services for Childbearing Women in Twentieth-Century Britain*. Oxford: Clarendon Press, pp. 30–46.

Pilley Edwards, N. (2005) *Birthing Autonomy Women's Experiences of Planning Home Births*. London: Routledge.

Potter, J. (1764) *Archaeologia Graeca (The Antiquities of Greece)*, Vol. II, pp. 324–5.

Robinson, S. (1990) Maintaining the independence of the midwifery profession; a continuing struggle. In Garcia, J. Kilpatrick, R. Richards, M. (eds.) *The Politics of Maternity Care: Services for Childbearing Women in Twentieth Century Britain*. Oxford: Clarendon Press, pp. 47–91.

Sharp, J. (1671) *The Midwives Book*. London: Simon Miller. New edition with introductory notes and commentary by Hobby, E. (ed.) (1999) *The Midwives Book*. Oxford: Oxford University Press.

Shelton, D.C. (2010) The emperor's new clothes. *Journal of the Royal Society of Medicine*, 103, 46–50.

Tew, M. (1998) *Safer Childbirth? A Critical History of Maternity Care*, 3rd edn. London: Free Association Books.

Towler, J. and Bramall, J. (1986) *Midwives in History and Society*. London: Croom Helm.

Van Gennep, A. (2004) *The Rites of Passage*. London: Routledge & Kegan Paul.

Walsh, D. (2007) *Evidence-Based Care for Normal Labour and Birth: A Guide for Midwives*. London: Routledge.

Wesson, N. (2006) *Home Birth: A Practical Guide*, 4th edn. London: Pinter & Martin.

Chapter 2   **Choosing homebirth**

Julia Magill-Cuerden

Introduction

Focusing on advice and information, this chapter considers planning and decision-making made by women when opting for homebirth. The views of women are largely ignored in the debate about homebirth (Jannsen *et al.*, 2009) and women are often not informed about the facilities available (Edwards, 2005). The discussion below provides advice and information for planning birth at home with guidance on the effects of the environment and safety considerations.

Informing women

Prior to informing women about the place of birth and having a homebirth, it is essential that midwives, and indeed other professionals, recognise the right of all women to give birth in a place of their choosing (Nursing and Midwifery Council, 2006, 2009a).

The right to choice of place of birth

This right to choose where to have a baby has been clearly promoted in government documents and statutory bodies over the last decade (House of Commons, 1992, 2003; Department of Health, 1993, 2000, 2004, 2007; Welsh Assembly Government, 2002, 2005; NHS Scotland, 2003; Department of Health and Department for Education and Skills, 2004; Nursing and Midwifery Council, 2006; and the NHS Choices website) and by women's groups (Association for Improvements in Maternity Services, undated; National Childcare Trust website). It is implicit in the midwives' code (Nursing and Midwifery Council, 2008) and *Midwives Rules and Standards* (Nursing and Midwifery Council, 2004).

The idea of choice encompasses more than just decision-making, with its implication that the onus is on a woman to opt for one choice; choice arises when a woman is able to make decisions based on information and support provided by professionals who are assisting in planning her care (Department of Health, 2007, p. 5). The information provided by midwives should be evidence based. If women have a right to choose their birthing place, then all women have a right to have a homebirth (Beech, 2004). Women may be referred to the homebirth website (BirthChoices UK). Friends and family may also influence a woman in her choices and her levels of anxiety (Barnett *et al.*, 2008), including her partner's view of infant rearing (Davies, 2008; see the Fatherhood Institute, n.d.). A midwife may assist by meeting partners and close family relatives prior to the birth or through preparation for labour classes to provide realistic support.

Prior to making any choice, it is imperative that women fully understand the implications and outcomes of decision-making and that professionals respect their dignity and individual requirements (Nursing and Midwifery Council, 2004, 2008). Offering guidance on best options available may allow plans to be flexible, leaving final decisions until the time of birth.

Services in local areas, which vary across the country, may influence decision-making for birth plans. Women should be advised to investigate the services offered locally and discuss these with their midwife. If necessary, a woman may need to talk to the commissioners for local healthcare services from their local primary care trust (NHS Choices website). Professionals need to be mindful that women have a right to refuse care and this applies to receiving care in hospital (Nursing and Midwifery Council, 2008); however, it is essential to ensure that women understand the implications of any actions they decide to take.

Decision-making may also be influenced by family beliefs, culture, background and personal values (Edwards, 2005). Because in parts of the world homebirth is not an option for maternity care, women's decisions may result from their social and cultural experiences (Sookhoo, 2009); therefore, birthing within the family and social circle may be seen as inappropriate and may be considered unsafe and a medical event (Edwards, 2005).

All health professionals need to examine their own attitudes towards homebirth as personal views and beliefs may influence the information they provide. Two studies demonstrate that midwives play an important part in influencing women in making a decision to have a homebirth (Wiegers *et al.*, 2000; Jannsen *et al.*, 2009). The values and beliefs of midwives may be influenced by their personal background; thus, professionals, by their own attitude and behaviour, may create a negative approach to homebirth (Thomas, 1998). Developing a culture so that midwives offer unbiased information requires professional development and training. Midwives should also be aware that a negative attitude towards homebirth may be reflected in their communications with women (Department of Health, 1993; Chamberlain *et al.*, 1997; Edwards, 2005; Madden, 2005; Stephens, 2005).

The final decisions about where to give birth rests with the mother, who as an individual determines her own care (Beech, 2004). The responsibility of healthcare professionals is to ensure that their advice to each woman results in women understanding the actions and the implications of any choices made (Dimond, 2006).

What advice and information

Full information and implications of this option of individually birthing at home should be given to *all* women (Dimond, 2006; National Midwifery Council, 2006, 2008). In a study carried out in 2000, many women reported that they did not receive this information but would have liked to do so, along with appropriate support (Singh and Newburn, 2000).

Midwives should discuss the best options, tailoring advice for each woman so that it takes into account her specific history and background, based on her knowledge and experience. Ideally each maternity unit will have a policy for homebirth.

In providing information the midwife has a statutory duty to provide professional care and practice based on the advice (National Midwifery Council, 2004, 2008), taking the woman's background into consideration, as shown in Table 2.1. She will also consider the practical midwifery issues.

Practical midwifery issues

GENERAL HISTORY OF THE WOMAN

It is essential to have full picture of the woman's health, as in routine pregnancy care: observation will be made of overall general health, height, weight, and information on any disability. Women with some types of disability, for example blindness, may labour more easily in a familiar environment, that is, disability should not be a barrier to homebirth provided the disability is not likely to impede a normal birth. A full routine health check should be completed. Planning for a homebirth is based on the assumption that the woman has no health conditions that would pose a risk. This will need to

TABLE 2.1 Background areas for a midwife to consider when advising a woman on homebirth

---

Cultural and personal issues
Beliefs for her personal care and that of her baby
Her knowledge of homebirth
Her emotional requirements for her birth and if birthing at home will accommodate this
Her psychological view of birthing and having a baby
Cultural acceptability of homebirth (van der Hulst *et al.*, 2004)
View of her partner and family on birth at home

---

be discussed at the first antenatal visit and the woman advised that, should a health problem arise during pregnancy, medical opinion would be sought for the implications in continuing with plans for homebirth.

PERSONAL WISHES FOR HER BIRTH

A midwife will need to discover if women view homebirth as normal as this may reflect their expectations of childbirth. A small study in The Netherlands found that women who are receptive to technology in the process of childbirth are more likely to opt for hospital birth (van der Hulst *et al.*, 2004). These authors suggest that women's perceptions and expectations influence their decisions on place of birth.

Birth is often perceived by women to be fraught with problems and messy. Midwives may explain the statistics of birthing at home where careful planning has taken place (Olsen, 1997; National Perinatal Epidemiology Unit, 2010). An explanation of the equipment used and precautions taken by the midwife should mitigate fears.

FAMILY AND SOCIAL CIRCUMSTANCES

Discovering the kinds of support that are likely to be available to a woman in labour is necessary. A partner or close family or friend present at birth who has a negative view of homebirth may influence women's feelings of comfort in the home environment. The midwife may offer to meet with partners and family to explain birthing at home or offer alternative plans, such as labouring early at home with decisions made to transfer to hospital, as necessary, once labour is established. It is important for women to feel confident in their decisions.

HER MEDICAL HISTORY

Details of any medical or health problems and how these are managed are essential. Not all conditions exclude birth at home, but it is important to ensure that any condition is stabilised prior to delivery. It may be important, in the case of women with psychological problems, such as a phobia of hospitals, that homebirth is an option. However, in this circumstance it would be essential for the midwife to make an arrangements for the woman to visit the maternity unit and meet the staff for orientation and in case of a emergency transfer to hospital. Details such as this must be recorded, with the woman's permission, in the records so that other staff offer appropriate care.

HER OBSTETRIC HISTORY

A detailed history of any previous births, that is, a full obstetric history, including place of birth and obstetric problems, is essential. The midwife should also obtain and scrutinise the notes pertaining to previous deliveries. For example, with a history of previous forceps delivery, it is prudent to determine the type of delivery and why forceps were used. If there is a history of caesarean section, the midwife should investigate why this was performed to determine whether there is a risk, in a future pregnancy, that the fetus might have difficulty traversing the birth canal. If a caesarean section was necessary because of cephalopelvic disproportion, for example, then any future birth needs to take place adjacent to an obstetric theatre. However, if the reason for the caesarean was fetal distress, then the cause should be investigated although there may be no evidence to suggest that this is likely to recur. Advisedly, medical opinion should be sought.

If a woman has a history of rapid deliveries it may be preferable to plan for a home delivery and ensure that all midwives within the team are aware of the history. If this is the case, it could also be useful to plan with the paramedical team in case of an emergency.

USE OF EVIDENCE AND RESEARCH

For those who request homebirth with a medical or obstetric condition with obvious contraindications for normal birthing, the midwife may find it useful to search for evidence and share this with the woman. The midwife is in the best position to advise women and identify rigorous evidence against opinion-related information.

When meeting a woman from early pregnancy onwards, midwives may assess issues that influence appropriate decisions when opting for homebirth. For example, those who wish to ensure total relief of pain or opt for an epidural will not be suitable candidates for initially planning a homebirth. However, attitudes and beliefs may change during pregnancy or labour; thus, flexibility in providing information about homebirth initially may assist women in their thinking. The midwife needs to be sensitive to a woman changing her mind and her wishes.

EMOTIONAL EXPECTATIONS

Whilst attitudes may influence choices about place of birth, eliciting the emotional views of women towards their birth affects decision-making. A midwife using her knowledge and experience in supporting women creates emotional bonds in the relationship during the process of birth (Wilkins, 2000).

Homebirth provides women with a greater sense of:

- empowerment (Janssen *et al.*, 2009; Morison *et al.*, 1998);
- self-confidence (Janssen *et al.*, 2009);
- bonding with the baby – this occurs earlier (Kitzinger, 1979);
- trust in the midwife (Janssen *et al.*, 2009);
- satisfaction with the birth in home or home-like settings (Hodnett *et al.*, 2005; Christiaens and Bracke, 2009).

The baby immediately adapts to a family environment when birth takes place at home (Boucher *et al.*, 2009). Suggested benefits of homebirth are shown in Table 2.2.

TABLE 2.2 Suggested benefits of homebirth

Benefit	Source of information
Physical	
Lower intervention rates	National Institute for Health and Clinical Excellence (2007), Boucher *et al.* (2009)
Fewer induced labours	National Institute for Health and Clinical Excellence (2007)
Fewer augmented labours	National Institute for Health and Clinical Excellence (2007)
Reduced use of epidural analgesia	National Institute for Health and Clinical Excellence (2007)
Women less likely to use drugs for pain relief	Chamberlain *et al.* (1997)
Lower rate of caesarean section	National Institute for Health and Clinical Excellence (2007)
Fewer episiotomies	National Institute for Health and Clinical Excellence (2007)
Lower incidence of infection	Janssen *et al.* (2009)
Psychological	
Feeling in control	Boucher *et al.* (2009) Andrews (2004a,b)[a]
Neonatal	
Baby alert	Andrews (2004a,b)[a]
Baby calm	Andrews (2004a,b)[a]

a   Taken from a small study of birthing exploring a planned homebirth.

CONTINUITY OF CARER WHEN BIRTHING AT HOME

Women who birth at home are more likely to receive care from a midwife they know and the midwife is more likely to remain for the duration of the labour, providing continuity of carer (Chamberlain *et al.*, 1997). Therefore, it is important that women have the opportunity during their pregnancy to meet all the midwives in the team who may be their carers. Continuity of carer, particularly in labour, provides empowerment for women.

At all times the midwife must remember that she is a guest in the house of the family and the woman is the hostess. If a woman is confident she will be more likely to be in control and feel relaxed and stress free (Chamberlain *et al.*, 1997; Macfarlane *et al.*, 2000).

GIVING ADVICE AND INFORMATION

Women who birth at home or in hospital require antenatal education and preparation for labour (Nolan *et al.*, 2009a). Similarly, they will require information about useful and informative websites and sources that offer the best and evidence-based information (Nolan *et al.*, 2009b).

The ability to provide unbiased advice and knowledge depends upon the individual. Personal beliefs need to be set aside. Where there is evidence this should be provided, offering the parameters surrounding the interpretation of that evidence, in relation to the woman's circumstances and through judicious use of the experience of the midwife (Sackett *et al.*, 2000; Gray, 2001).

Communicating information

Communicating information for homebirth is multifaceted, and Chamberlain and colleagues (1997, p. 234), in their homebirth study, suggested that it should be 'understandable, accurate, in the language and syntax that is acceptable to recipients, reflect local facilities and practices'.

Providing advice appropriate to every situation is an art and skill based on knowledge and experience. The art lies in knowing how to interpret the information, in relation to each individual and taking into consideration their social and cultural background. The skill is in *how* this is communicated verbally and non-verbally. We are not all successful at this, and most of us, when offering information, have at some point failed to be clearly understood by the receiver. Help may be required from other people to communicate in a different way for appropriate comprehension. Communication exchanges depend upon verbal (language skills) and non-verbal skills being in tandem with each other, and confidence in the knowledge imparted and the ability of the woman and her partner to interpret communications and signals given. Similarly, the midwife must comprehend expressions and language by women.

The use of interpreters is encouraged when women do not converse confidently in English. Family members and partners should not be used for discussions as confidentiality must be respected (National Midwifery Council, 2008). However, in a home situation the midwife may need to plan with the family for use of a suitable person as an interpreter who would be acceptable to both the woman and the midwife. A high quality of communication is central to the provision of maternity care (Homeyard and Gaudion, 2008).

Giving information with sensitivity

A final choice for place of birth may not necessarily take place until the woman is in labour, though this may be influenced by local policy schemes (National Midwifery Council, 2006). In discussion about the information for homebirth, women need to be made aware of:

* the local NHS trust's policy on homebirth;
* the criteria for having a birth at home (this may be indicative but midwives need to use their assessment of each woman with her views of birthing at home).

Suggesting to women that they prepare a written plan for discussion with the midwife is useful for birthing either at home or another venue (National Midwifery Council, 2006) and it encourages women to think about their choices (Hollis Martin, 2008). Having a written plan enables midwives to exchange information regarding the woman's wishes around issues such as pain relief, attendees at birth, technology usage and gender of attendee at birth, all which can aid continuity of care. A useful website for women to access when planning care is NHS Choices (NHS Choices: Your Health, Your Choices), which has a 'Where to Give Birth' page. A plan, used effectively, also allows a retrospective review for evaluating the birth, enabling women to identify highlights and disappointments in their birth (Hollis Martin, 2008). A midwife may explain occurrences, dispel myths or allay anxieties that may result later or in subsequent pregnancies.

Who attends the birth?

The midwives who attend the birth, whether known or one of a team, or a professional to whom the woman has not been introduced, need to be aware of all the options of care discussed in pregnancy. The personal knowledge of the woman by the midwife affects a woman's view of the professional supporting her during birthing at home (BirthChoiceUK website).

When to inform women

Ideally, options for care should be discussed at the first booking visit (House of Commons, 2004). At no stage during her pregnancy should any pressure be placed on women to make choices regarding the place of birth (House of Commons, 2004). During the antenatal period, the discussion of homebirth may be raised at any time. It is good practice to record in the antenatal notes when types of options for birth have been discussed. This will ensure that none of the full range of options is forgotten.

As there is so much information to be imparted to women at the first antenatal visit, it may be helpful for some discussions to be held at a later visit for full explanation. Many women are not aware that they may change their mind as their pregnancy progresses and this point needs to be brought to their attention. They may subsequently opt for a homebirth. Therefore, returning to discuss this option throughout pregnancy provides optimum choice.

When women are referred by a midwife or GP to hospital for a medical opinion, there is often a single flow of direction for women; they may remain under hospital care as if, by default, they should be considered only for hospital care. When a woman attends hospital for further (medical) opinion she should be debriefed by the midwife who has referred her, in a full discussion that enables women to share their understanding and experiences and to have their views recognised. Further plans for the future pregnancy and birth will take into consideration the advice and any treatment provided as well as the woman's wishes. This provides continuity of care (Edwards, 2005). Midwives need to ensure that women's preferences are still respected in spite of changes in circumstances and that they fully understand all the implications of any changes.

At around 36 weeks the midwife should visit the woman at home to discuss plans for birthing at home. Although this time is not prescriptive, it precedes 37 weeks' gestation, when a normal birth is more likely. After this time, it may be too late for the event and to put in place appropriate preparations. Both the role of the midwife in undertaking her professional duties and the role of the woman with her preparation responsibilities should be clear and fully understood. This planning assists women to take control of their own event of birth. It is important to ensure that the woman's supporting partner does not have other duties, such as caring for other children. In case of an emergency there must be one responsible adult available in the home to assist and to call for medical aid. The preparations at this visit include a full explanation of details given in Table 2.3.

TABLE 2.3 Details and discussion around 36 weeks' gestation

Equipment to be obtained by the mother

Water pool if required

Lighting

Music

Waterproof protection for mattress, if used, or for the floor

Baby equipment – clothes, cot, linen, towels

Home heating in summer and winter

Equipment to be obtained by the midwife – see chapters 4 and 5

Homebirth delivery pack (to be discussed)

Entonox equipment

Oxygen

Suturing equipment

Emergency equipment, such as intravenous fluids

Drugs such as Syntocinon

Information to be discussed

Preparation for labour and delivery

Pain relief: obtaining drugs and equipment, for example, that the midwife will bring
or the women needs to obtain

Role of supporters in labour

Fluids and diet in labour

Getting the home ready for the birth

Where to be in the house during labour and delivery

Water birth, pool and equipment, if required

Where to put the baby after birth (cot, clothes, review warm and non-draughty areas
in cold weather, baby bath and so forth)

Practical information

Protection of the home furnishings

Disposal of the placenta

Informing the midwife of labour

How to call the midwife

Which midwife to call

When to call the midwife when in labour, for example when there is a show,
ruptured membranes or regular rhythmic contractions

Midwifery care and the process of birth

Assistance and support in labour (review antenatal preparation)

Rehearse positions for labour

Midwifery requirement to take observations and make records of progress in labour

TABLE **2.3** (continued)

Attending midwifery staff at birth (students, midwifery or medical, other midwives, such as health care assistant)

Role of doula (a formalised arrangement for a birth companion), if arranged

Social care

Ideally, for one adult person at home who will be available at all times for the midwife and who is not involved with care of other people or children

Child care

Other members of the family and friends at home

Birth partner and family support (roles in labour)

Support in early labour

Support when labour established

Calling the midwife

Use of a card/leaflet with all the numbers, including midwife, labour ward and supervisor of midwives contacts

The midwife's role when called

Her anticipated support in early labour

Her support when labour established

Early labour and false labour

Emergency information (in pregnancy or labour or after birth)

If emergency arises prior to labour when and how to call the midwife (telephone number of midwife and others to be called)

Discuss likely emergencies, for example sudden bleeding, reduced or loss of fetal movement, acute and prolonged pain

The hospital number in case of need

Information about an unexpected need to go into hospital during the birth

How to obtain assistance in an emergency during labour or delivery

Situations that might occur when labour is established or during delivery for the woman to be transferred into hospital, for example if vaginal bleeding occurs, first or second stage of labour is delayed, or there is fetal distress

---

Although friends and family may attend the birth to provide support, the woman's wishes for her birth should be respected (National Midwifery Council, 2008). Only people who are acceptable to her should be present during her birthing. Whereas the woman herself should be in control of who is present for her birth and supporting her, the midwife must be present for monitoring the progress of labour and for delivery (National Midwifery Council, 2004). The midwife is accountable for all her actions as if she were attending any birth. She must ensure that appropriate observations and recordings are made and that these are discussed.

Low-risk women

Using the terminology of 'risk' is problematic and the idea of 'low risk' is itself dubious and complex. Indeed, the concept of placing women in different categories of being 'at risk' is also problematic (see Walsh, 2003) as we then place women into boxes. Although the use of the terms 'low risk' and 'high risk' is commonplace in midwifery and obstetrics, each woman's circumstances must be reflected in the care provided. For example, a woman who has poor social circumstances but a fear of hospital may better be cared for at home rather than in hospital, where her fear may create the need for interventions. Through planning and remaining at home, non-interventionist care may be provided. Safe care is possible in varied environments, for example caravans, boats, tents or squatting houses, provided the principles of competent midwifery care are adhered to, the environment is hygienic, with access to water, a toilet and heating, and there is easy access for emergency services. The aim of a homebirth is to provide women who are expected to have a vaginal birth with the opportunity to deliver their baby in their home environment and within their social setting.

Homebirth and maternal physical well-being

Kitzinger (1979) stresses the importance of birthing in an environment within the social and family setting. We do not know the outcomes of different psychological effects of hospital birth and homebirthing on subsequent family and parental relationships. Nor is there evidence to indicate the effects of the environment on the physical abilities or the powers of the women to labour (Walsh *et al.*, 2004). The relationship between the psychology of the environment and hormonal functions is currently unknown. The outcomes of labour in many circumstances cannot be predicted (Walsh *et al.*, 2004), and evidence of the effects on women choosing to birth in a place where they are confident is not available. This reiterates a need for not confirming decisions about the place or a homebirth until the time of birth itself, where a non-interventionist birth is anticipated. Being flexible about where birth takes place enables decisions to be made optimally for each woman.

Although an NHS trust may lay down eligibility criteria, this information provides a basis for a guidance and discussion. During a pregnancy the woman's condition may change. Therefore, any final decision may be unsuitable at an early stage in pregnancy.

Homebirth and psychological and emotional health

The opportunity for homebirth increases the possibility of continuity of care (Edwards, 2005). Continuous carer support has been shown to have meaningful benefits, such as promoting vaginal birth (Hodnett *et al.*, 2011).

Midwives build particular relationships with women in labour, which Holloway and Bluff (1994) and Wilkins (2000) consider special. The individual or special relationship occurs when both hold similar values. This assists women to gain in confidence in their birth (Morison *et al.*, 1999). 'Trust' relationships are formed and this relationship is built from women's confidence in their birthing experience (Wilkins, 2000; Edwards, 2005). However, Morison and colleagues (1999) suggest that where similar beliefs are not held there is potential for conflict. This indicates that midwives need to be fully aware of women's personal values for their birth to provide support for personal expectations.

Women who opt for homebirth may wish to retain control and value the emotional safety of their own environment (Walsh *et al.*, 2004). Offering homebirth offers women who are anxious about being in hospital the safety of their own home; this reduces the anxiety–pain relationship (Escott *et al.*, 2004) and promotes normal birth (Royal College of Midwives, 2004).

Criteria for decisions of place of birth

Safety of homebirth

Absolute safety for women in birth cannot be assured at home, in a midwifery-led unit or in hospital, and all places may have risks attached. The risks involved in birthing at home need to be balanced with those of delivering in other venues, such as a hospital. Currently, there is little reliable evidence to compare the safety of homebirth with birth in a hospital or in a midwifery-led unit where a non-interventionist outcome is anticipated (National Perinatal Epidemiology Unit, 2010). A recent review of planned homebirth in the UK and overseas concluded that current evidence available does not support claims that hospital birth is safer than planned homebirth for women who have a healthy 'straightforward pregnancy' (Gyte and Dodwell, 2008, p. 384). The benefits of labouring and birthing in both places require discussion with women to ensure working in partnership (International Confederation of Midwives, 2005).

Using evidence and research to define 'safety' promotes the notion that 'risk' is central to maternity care and its outcomes. However, caution is required in using these terms as neither is an absolute concept and both may be interpreted by individual women and midwives according to their personal values. Safety does not necessarily encompass technology that may under-value skills and judgements made by the midwife using her personal skills, emotional and midwifery support of labouring women (Edwards, 2008). The term 'safety' may mean more to a woman than having an outcome of a healthy baby. It may mean maintaining self-worth and self-esteem (Edwards, 2008). Therefore, the advice given is dependent upon the interpretation of evidence for that particular woman in her individual circumstances.

From studies over the last few decades it appears that when the profile of a woman is suitable and with an anticipated outcome of normal birth, the perinatal hazards of homebirth are low and mostly unavoidable (Northern Region Perinatal Mortality Survey Coordinating Group, 1996). This finding is supported by a meta-analysis of international studies by Olsen (1997), who found little difference between homebirth and hospital birth perinatal mor-tality rates. Although Campbell and Macfarlane (1994) suggest that rates of maternal morbidity are lower at home, they did not compare homebirth with births in midwifery-led units attached to hospitals and their figures are not based on current evidence.

When discussing homebirth with women, midwives should be aware of the differences between planned homebirth and a baby born before arrival (BBA). Many figures for homebirth include BBAs and, therefore, confuse the statis-tics; however, there is no national definition of this term, and some women who plan a homebirth have been recorded as a BBA (Ford and Pett, 2008). In the homebirth study, unplanned homebirths or BBAs were found to be associ-ated with a higher level of perinatal morbidity and mortality (Chamberlain *et al.*, 1997).

Criteria for homebirth

Many units provide written lists or criteria for offering homebirth although there is little evidence of who will birth well or not so well at home and there does not appear to be a consensus for specific criteria. Campbell (1999) found that criteria for each NHS trust were based on obstetric and midwifery opinion. Table 2.4 outlines suggested criteria.

Campbell (1999) suggests that using criteria has the potential to label women with risk categories and is, therefore, discriminatory and reduces women's choices and options. However, the 2002–3 Confidential Enquiry into Maternal and Child Health (CEMACH, 2005) report suggests that midwives should have clear risk assessment criteria for homebirth and that care should be planned individually (CEMACH-CEMACE, 2007); thus, midwives should give careful consideration to the situation for each woman when interpreting

TABLE **2.4** Suggested outline criteria for use to identify women suitable for homebirth following the study by Janssen and colleagues (2009)

Singleton pregnancy

Cephalic presentation

No pre-existing medical disorders, such as diabetes, cardiac disorder or renal disease

Absence of pregnancy-related disorders, such as placenta praevia, pregnancy bleeding, pregnancy-induced hypertension with proteinuria or active genital herpes

Absence of malpresentation

---

criteria. When conflict arises between the criteria and women's choices, it is good practice for the midwife to seek her manager's or supervisor of midwives' assistance and that he or she also meets with both the woman and the midwife.

High-risk women

Women who are likely to have birth complications and who wish for homebirth should be fully informed of the current evidence available regarding their condition, including the outcomes and possibilities should the woman decide to deliver at home. All medical referrals from the midwife should be to senior members of the medical team.

Options for care

Every woman should be offered the full range of different options for delivery to accommodate her wishes. For example:

- remaining at home until labour is established or until a medical problem indicates the need for transfer;
- arranging for minimal time in hospital with early transfer home planned;
- being cared for within a midwifery-led unit should labour commence normally and where transfer may be made easily to an obstetric consultant unit;
- receiving total care for labour and delivery in a hospital environment and maybe early arrangement for transfer home.

Women need to be aware of the best practices available for their situations. Any risks must be explained using evidence. Should the woman require an epidural for a medical or obstetric condition then her option is to be cared for in hospital. Similarly, if monitoring or surveillance of, or advice about, the progress of labour is required for either mother or fetus by a team because of a medical or obstetric condition, then she will most advisedly receive care in a hospital setting with appropriate facilities. It has been shown that where there are indecisions in planning a transfer, the maternal and perinatal outcomes are poorer (Chamberlain *et al.*, 1997).

If a woman is considered to have a condition that is likely to necessitate interventions during her birthing or medical or obstetric care and wishes to birth at home, her options need to be discussed fully, including possible outcomes. This is where looking at all the evidence and sharing the implications with women is the initial first line of practice. Honesty and openness is essential and advice should not be based on opinions that are not supported by evidence. Where the outcome is unknown, the problems associated with this should be made clear. For example, if a woman who has had a previous caesarean section wishes her next birth to be at home, then it is important to discover the reasons for the caesarean section. If this was for fetal distress and during this pregnancy there are no likely problems but expectations are for a normal birth outcome, the midwife might consider looking at vaginal birth after caesarean section (VBAC) literature and evidence with the woman and discuss the possible implications of delivering at home.

If, however, the fetal distress occurred after long delay in labour and the previous birth was considered prolonged labour, then it would be preferable to be in hospital for the birth of this next baby in case of recurrence. In these cases the midwife should be clear in informing women and recording the likely outcomes of her decisions and actions.

Should a decision be made for a homebirth where there has been a complication of present or previous pregnancy, it would be prudent for the woman to visit an obstetrician during pregnancy to review the feasibility of a normal birth. It would be useful to discuss this with the supervisor of midwives, who could also review the past and present history with the woman and review the options for birth. There are several possible outcomes:

- Labour care and birthing could be arranged in a midwifery-led unit adjacent to a hospital unit where normality could be anticipated unless problems occur from the outset of labour. Transfer to the hospital facilities can then take place with ease.
- The midwife who would have been attendant at the homebirth could provide continuity of care in labour in the hospital.
- When labour commences the woman may initially labour at home but with the labour ward informed provided a member of the midwifery team can provide early home support. Transfer may be facilitated once it is deemed no longer suitable to labour at home.

Each of these options would require a specific birth plan discussed with the woman so that she and her family are able to consider the pathways to take if necessary. Should a woman with a likely complication opt for a homebirth prior going into labour the correct procedure is as follows:

- The midwife should inform her manager or supervisor of midwives, who will, ideally, make a home visit providing advice on best evidence and the likely outcome at birth. It is the supervisor of midwives' role to support both the woman and the midwife (Nursing and Midwifery Council, 2009a). It is good practice for the supervisor of midwives to make a home visit with the midwife and review the circumstances in detail. The supervisor of midwives will also assist in communications with the medical staff, the midwifery managers and the midwife.
- The midwife should ensure that arrangements are in place for emergency transfer to hospital if necessary. This would include alerting the emergency ambulance team so they are aware of both the situation and the residential address.
- The supervisor of midwives will alert the supervisory team so that a supervisor of midwives is available at all times during the period that the woman is likely to go into labour to provide advice to the midwife. Ideally, this will be to support and assist the woman in her choices.

Care against medical and midwifery advice

Should this event occur, the supervisor of midwives, midwifery manager and midwife will need to agree a plan of care with the woman. Good practice will enable all to meet to put in place a documented plan of care. Communications need to be made with labour ward and hospital team to prepare for any transfer. When the woman goes into labour and remains at home the supervisor of midwives on call should be contacted to provide support. It may be necessary for her to be present at the home. It is also advisable, at this time, to keep in close up-to-date contact with the medical staff so that advice may be sought early and that all parties are fully informed. This will be explained to the woman. Good practice would be to write a plan of care for each person to follow.

Should the woman not agree to a plan of care that has been devised, the midwifery team may find it helpful to have options written and agreed by all those involved in the care, and the woman should be made aware of its existence, although she has a right to disagree. The midwife is pivotal in maintaining good communications and relationships with the woman.

Midwives should not undertake any practice that compromises their professional actions for safe care. Though a midwife cannot refuse to provide care, her accountability for her own practice should be made clear to the woman (Nursing and Midwifery Council, 2006). The midwife should seek advice from the supervisor of midwives on call if she has any concerns. Although a midwife or other professional cannot refuse to comply with a woman who decides to give birth at home and may disagree with the choices the woman has made, she must still provide unbiased support and care to the woman. The woman must be fully informed about the options as a result of any actions taken (Nursing and Midwifery Council, 2004, 2008). It is essential that full documentation is completed (Nursing and Midwifery Council, 2009b).

It is important for the midwife to recognise her professional responsibility only to provide safe care (Nursing and Midwifery Council, 2008). If a woman requests care that the midwife considers unsafe, the midwife must give reasons and explanations and record this fully in the notes and ask the woman to read her recording. However, whatever the woman's decision, the midwife's role is to support the mother (Nursing and Midwifery Council, 2009a). Should she not agree with the woman's decisions, she should contact her manager and/or the supervisor of midwives for advice, see the woman and discuss the situation. The midwife should not put her own safety, or her professional accountability, in jeopardy.

Where a woman's condition is such that the birth should take place in hospital, the midwife should bear in mind that the relationships between anxiety and fear lead to higher levels of tension and pain (Escott *et al.*, 2004). Therefore, discovering a reason for fears and attempting to mitigate these may be a priority (see Table 2.5).

TABLE 2.5 Examples of fear of being admitted to hospital care

Fear of needles
Fear of being placed under a mask
Fear of the smell of hospitals
Associating hospital with the place of death of loved ones or of dying
Previous poor obstetric experience or obstetric experience resulting in post-traumatic stress disorder
Fear of authority and recognition by the state surveillance systems, particularly in the case of refugees or migrants
Anxiety of leaving other children at home and violence in the family
Fear of social services intervention in the home circumstances

Where possible, the midwife should seek, with the woman, to find solutions to provide the best possible care. It may be necessary for the midwife to accompany the woman on all visits to medical staff, to intercede for her in conversations, acting as an advocate, and seek the most appropriate solution for care. A supervisor of midwives can assist with this.

Transfer

The likelihood of end-pregnancy or intrapartum transfer to hospital must be discussed with all women who plan to deliver at home so that the possibility is recognised (Department of Health, 1993). A recent review of intrapartum transfer found that the transfer from home to hospital rate varies from 7.4 to 16.5 per cent (Fullerton *et al.*, 2007). The evidence of outcomes following transfer is variable across the country (National Institute for Health and Clinical Evidence, 2008). Women may require time to reflect upon the impact of this emergency, were it to happen, and the impact on their family (Department of Health, 1993).

Evidence of this discussion should be recorded in the notes for interprofessional communication. Although the idea should be introduced in pregnancy, detailed discussion takes place at the 36-week visit. Leaving a discussion of the possibility of transfer until late in pregnancy or during labour may cause conflict when it has not been an anticipated occurrence. The woman, her partner and her family should be made fully aware of smooth management and their responsibilities, such as:

- assistance with phoning;
- ensuring directions to the home are correct;
- ensuring facilities are available for emergency transport to access the home (with lighting at night);
- caring for other children in this situation (Warwick, 2004).

Chamberlain and colleagues (1997) found that less favourable outcomes were associated with transfer in labour to hospital during delivery a first baby, especially when continuity of carer was absent, and they suggested that outcomes could be improved by better communication between community and hospital teams. CEMACH-CEMACE (2007) emphasises the need for good communication between home and hospital staff. The midwife transferring the woman should communicate directly with a senior member of the obstetric team. Once a transfer has taken place, the hospital team should respect her report.

When transfer to hospital occurs, the midwife attending her at home is invaluable in providing continuity of care and also in acting as the advocate of the woman when in a different environment (Edwards, 2005). This is a unique role in mediating women's wishes when expectations have changed. This is more easily managed when community midwives work in both the hospital and the community, but women should be advised that it may not be possible for a midwife to remain with her for the duration of labour.

Furthermore, the midwife, through building up a relationship of trust, needs to ensure that the woman's wishes do not compromise her paramount role of safe practice (Nursing and Midwifery Council, 2008).

It can be helpful for a woman to visit the hospital during pregnancy, meet the labour ward staff and become familiar with the building environment and facilities in case of immediate of emergency care. This may mitigate some of the anxiety caused should a transfer be required.

Resources to support homebirth

A homebirth leaflet provides advice for women which may be used for discussion with families and partners and to ensure they are aware of their responsibilities when birthing at home. Suggestions for inclusion in a leaflet for homebirth are given in Table 2.6.

This leaflet could be designed to form a contract between midwife and woman where specific details are documented if these are not included in the notes.

Place of delivery

Discussion takes place between the woman and midwife as to the best place in her home for labour and birthing the baby. Some women prefer to have the birth in the main living room, and this may be where a water pool may

TABLE 2.6 Information leaflet: suggested areas for inclusion

Responsibilities of the midwife
Responsibilities of the woman
Responsibilities of the family and supporting friends
How to contact the midwife and supervisor of midwives
How to contact the hospital or community service
What to do in an emergency when in the home or when travelling

be used for labour, pain relief or birthing. Women may prefer their own bath for use of pain relief in early labour. If the pool is to be used in a room that is not on the ground floor, then the householder should confirm that there is adequate support for the weight of water in the pool and that the room joists will hold.

During labour the woman may prefer to rest in her bed from time to time. The midwife and woman should discuss different positions, use of equipment such as a birth stool, and whether the woman would prefer to be on a bed or on a mattress or birthmat on the floor, with rehearsal of alternative positions to ensure manoeuvrability in the home. When in labour the woman will then be aware of positions. The midwife's responsibility is to ensure that a woman does not put unnecessary stress on her back by adopting awkward positions. If necessary, the bed may be raised on blocks for ease of care.

Lighting

During labour and birth dimmed lighting may be preferred. The midwife should determine that there is adequate lighting in the planned delivery area to visualise the perineum after delivery or if necessary for resuscitation or viewing the baby at birth.

Protective care

A midwife needs to advise a woman and her partner in advance about what protective covering may be useful to ensure that any furniture, bedding and flooring is protected. This is discussed at the antenatal visit.

People at delivery

The responsible adult available in the home during care in labour and birth should not have other responsibilities, such as care of the children, in case the midwife requires support or in an emergency. If children are present they will require a minder to ensure their care. Discussion needs to take place with the parents to ensure that they are prepared for the birth if they are to be present during the labour. During the earlier stages of labour the mother tends to be mobile and care of children takes place as normal. During birth only adults and children who have planned to be with the mother, with prior agreement, should attend the birth.

Place of equipment

It is useful for the midwife to have a specific flat surface or place to set out equipment in the area for giving birth. A place for the midwife to sit quietly in one area of the room may be helpful when labour is advancing, so that she can provide quiet but confident support.

Music or recording

Music assists peace and calm in labour. At all times the mother's wishes should be respected.

Professional staff resources

Providing homebirth is government policy and, should a midwife not be available to attend, this must be discussed with the supervisor of midwives. If necessary, the primary care trust that negotiates the contract for services should be involved. The maternity services are obliged to provide a midwife should a woman decide to birth at home and refuses to come into hospital (Beech, 2004). This problem should not occur with good planning and negotiation with women and families.

Professional at delivery

There is a requirement that the midwife or a medical professional is present at the birth (Midwives Act). It is incumbent upon the midwife to maintain the best possible relationship with the woman to ensure that a professional is present at the birth. Although there is no requirement to have more than one midwife during the later stages of labour and at delivery of the baby, it is usual to have two professional people available. This could be a student midwife or a responsible adult. It is important that the second person can assist with the resuscitation of the baby and provide support for the midwife. A second person is essential when emergencies arise to assist in gaining help.

Midwifery equipment

Most maternity units provide a 'homebirth pack', which will be taken to the woman's home at around 36 weeks. The pack contains a full set of equipment for delivery. When called for the delivery, the midwife will, in addition, need to take with her any drugs she requires. Table 2.7 gives a suggested list of additions to the list of equipment in Table 2.3. The midwife will have a full set

TABLE 2.7 Suggested equipment for a homebirth in addition to the equipment list in Table 2.3

Drugs including: a uterine-stimulating drug (3rd stage), an antidote to opioid drugs (if needed), an antiseptic, suturing material, local anaesthetic

Hand-held Pinard stethoscope and/or Sonicaid or other device for monitoring the fetal heartbeat

Sphygmomanometer

Adult stethoscope

---

of notes for labour and post delivery. Records should be maintained, as they would be in routine midwifery practice.

Medical back-up

Emergency communication must be considered for women in all stages of labour.

Ambulance and emergency services

The midwife must be familiar with the emergency numbers to contact, and these should be written and available for easy access should an emergency arise, so that any responsible adult may use them to convey any message. It is helpful for any messages to be written down (or dictated by the midwife for writing). Anxiety and stress may result in an inaccurate message in emergencies.

Should the midwife have any problems in providing care, or if conflict arises, she must contact the supervisor of midwives on call or the midwifery unit manager. Where emergency obstetric care is required, it could be helpful to speak directly to the senior obstetrician on call for the maternity unit. When calling the ambulance and emergency services the midwife should make it clear if an ambulance is required or a paramedical team at the home.

Safe birth environment

The midwife must ensure that her professional practice is in accordance with the contemporary standards for midwifery (Nursing and Midwifery Council, 2004).

Gaining skills and expertise

Once qualified, a midwife should be able to deliver a baby in any environment, in any position, and offer first aid care for obstetric or medical emergencies for both mother and baby (Nursing and Midwifery Council, 2006). However, on qualification she may not be fully conversant with these. It is, therefore, essential that all midwives ensure that they are fully equipped with these skills in the immediate post-qualifying period, prior to working in a home environment. Appropriate knowledge and skills may need to be adapted to the different environment (Department of Health, Social Services and Public Safety, 2000; Welsh Assembly Government, 2002; United Kingdom Parliament, 2004). Table 2.8 lists essential skills.

The midwife will also require training in essential skills in the wider role of the midwife as given in examples in Table 2.9. Additionally, a midwife will need to equip herself to undertake these procedures in a home environment; for example, if unexpectedly faced with any situation in Table 2.10 she should know how to manage this at home and know what to do whilst awaiting emergency for assistance *without having to rely on any other person*. She must be knowledgeable in these unexpected situations, however rare it is to encounter them.

Training should also be given in what should be avoided in homebirth, such as procedures that may lead to emergencies, for instance artificially rupturing the membranes.

TABLE 2.8 Knowledge and skills adaptation to the home environment

Creating a culture of calm and being non-obtrusive
Maintaining records contemporaneously
Monitoring the mother and fetus without being obtrusive
Use of different positions for birth and in different spaces
Use of water birth for labour and delivery
Contacting the supervisor of midwives
Contacting the labour ward and senior midwifery management

TABLE 2.9 Knowledge and skills required in the midwife's wider role to adapt to the home environment

Perineal suturing
Neonatal and adult resuscitation
Intravenous cannulation
Requesting emergency help and transfer from home to consultant unit
Assisting in water birth
District ambulance services (Department of Health, 1993)

TABLE 2.10 Emergencies requiring first aid training

Shoulder dystocia
Antenatal, intrapartum and postpartum haemorrhage
Cord prolapse
Breech presentations
Twin delivery, as an emergency situation
Malpresentations, for example face presentation
Prolonged labour and maternal distress
Obstructed labour
Fetal distress
Delay in the second stage of labour
Severe perineal trauma

Safety of the midwife

When making home visits midwives should ensure that they are familiar with the location and any hazards they might encounter in finding the home. Midwives have a duty to protect their own safety while locating the property and to make appropriate arrangements for transport of equipment and car parking. As the midwife is a visitor in the home of the clients she must take reasonable care for her own safety and to avoid damaging the property of others.

Negotiations may be necessary with the family to ensure safety, access and lighting for the midwife during the day, and particularly at night, and plans agreed between the midwifery team. The availability of secure parking needs to be confirmed prior to arriving for the delivery. Information about access must be conveyed to colleagues who may be required to attend the birth.

The midwife needs to ensure that the house is safe for her to enter and that she is not likely to injure herself; for example, she should check for unsafe stair carpets, floorboards and dim lighting where visibility is poor where care may be provided. Any safety concerns should be discussed with the supervisor of midwives and the maternity service provider.

Communication may be available through IT connections, mobile phones or internet, but not all places have, as yet, good connections. A landline may be necessary. Communications and contingency plans are essential in case of emergencies, particularly in inaccessible areas. Employers are responsible for ensuring the safety of their employees; therefore, midwives should inform the maternity unit of their whereabouts when attending a home (Royal College of Midwives, 2002). Midwives should take note of police warnings about theft and property damage and consider personal safety alarms.

Consideration needs to be given to access for lifting heavy equipment and emergency services in high-rise buildings. The number of lifts and stairways should be reviewed and discussed with the woman so that a working lift is accessible in emergencies. Similarly, in emergencies such as cord prolapse, the lift space may be required for a portable trolley for transfer of the woman (Richardson, 2009). The facilities may depend upon the level of floor; for example, a second- or third-floor stair access may be suitable in an emergency but an eighth or fourteenth floor may not be considered suitable.

Arrangements for the care of pets during labour and delivery should be considered and advice about pets, including dogs and cats, with newborn babies should be provided.

Conclusion

Women who receive the appropriate advice and information regarding the planned place of birth are likely to be satisfied with their care. The midwifery skills required to support homebirth may need to be adapted to the environment. The midwife and the woman frequently develop a special or emotional bond. Information given to women who wish to birth at home must be based on best available evidence. When providing advice and information, midwives should be conversant with their own training and development needs.

The importance of planning for a homebirth cannot be underestimated, and the midwife needs to ensure that each woman has an appropriate plan of care for her birth. With planning, risks may be avoided. Making sure that women are fully conversant with their progress in labour and their care needs, including the possibility of transfer to hospital, will reduce complications. Respecting the woman's choices may require careful negotiation and building up a special relationship of trust by the midwife. Providing advice and information honestly and without bias will enable the woman to make her own decisions for birthing at home.

References

Association for Improvements in Maternity Services (AIMS) (undated) *Choosing a Home Birth* (http://www.aims.org.uk/; accessed July 2010).

Andrews, A. (2004a) Home birth experience. 1. Decision and expectations. *British Journal of Midwifery*, 12, 518–23.

Andrews, A. (2004b) Home birth experience. 2. Births/postnatal reflections. *British Journal of Midwifery*, 12, 552–7.

Barnett, C., Hundley, V., Cheyne, H. and Kane, F. (2008) 'Not in labour': impact of sending women home in the latent phase. *British Journal of Midwifery*, 16, 144–3.

Beech, B. (2004) *Am I Allowed?* An Association for Improvements for Maternity Services (AIMS) publication. Surbiton, Surrey: BirthChoice UK (http://www.birthchoiceuk.com/; accessed June 2010).

Boucher, B., Bennett, C., Mcfarlin, B. and Freeze, R. (2009) Staying home to give birth: why women in the United States choose home birth. *Journal of Midwifery and Women's Health*, 54(2), 119–26.

Campbell, R. (1999) Review and assessment of selection criteria used when booking pregnant women at different places of birth. *British Journal of Obstetrics and Gynaecology*, 106, 550–6.

Campbell, R. and Macfarlane, A. (1994) *Where to Be Born: The Debate and the Evidence*, 2nd edn. Oxford: National Perinatal Epidemiology Unit.

Confidential Enquiry into Maternal and Child Health (CEMACH) (2005) *Why Mothers Die 2000–2002*. 6th Report. London: Royal College of Obstetricians and Gynaecologists Press.

Confidential Enquiry into Maternal and Child Health–Centre for Maternal and Child Enquiries, (CEMACH–CEMACE) (2007) *Saving Mother's Lives 2003–2005*. 7th Report. London: CEMACH.

Chamberlain, G., Wraight, A. and Crowley, P (1997) *Home Births*. London: Parthenon.

Christiaens, W. and Bracke, P. (2009) Place of birth and satisfaction with childbirth in Belgium and the Netherlands. *Midwifery*, 25(2), 11–19.

Davies, J. (2008) Completing the midwifery jigsaw. *Practising Midwife*, 11(11), 12–14.

Department of Health (1993) *Report of the Expert Group on the Maternity Service* (Changing Childbirth Report Part 1). London: Department of Health.

Department of Health (2000) *The NHS Plan*. Cmnd 481-81. London: The Stationery Office.

Department of Health (2004) *National Service Framework for Children, Young People and Maternity Services: Maternity Services*. Product No. 40498. London: Department of Health.

Department of Health (2007) *Maternity Matters: Choice, Access and Continuity of Care in a Safe Service*. London: Department of Health.

Department of Health and Department for Education and Skills (2004) *The National Service Framework for Children, Young People and the Maternity Services. Standard 11: Maternity Services*. London: Department of Health.

Department of Health, Social Services and Public Safety (2000) *The Contribution of Nurses, Midwives and Health Visitors: Valuing Diversity . . . A Way Forward*. Working Paper 2. Northern Ireland Department of Health, Social Services and Public Safety.

Dimond, B. (2006) *Legal Aspects of Midwifery*, 3rd edn. Edinburgh: Books for Midwives, Elsevier.

Edwards, N.P. (2005) *Birthing Autonomy: Women's Experiences of Planning Home Births*. London: Routledge.

Edwards, N. (2008) Safety in birth: the contextual conundrums faced by women in a 'risk society', driven by neoliberal policies. *MIDIRS Midwifery Digest*, 18, 463–70.

Escott, D., Spiby, H., Slade, P. and Fraser, R.B. (2004) The range of coping strategies women use to manage pain and anxiety prior to and during first experience of labour. *Midwifery*, 20, 144–56.

Fatherhood Institute (n.d.) http://www.fatherhoodinstitute.org/index.php?id=2&cID=578 (accessed July 2010).

Ford, J. and Pett, G. (2008) 'BBA' birth: analysis of one year's 'born before arrival' births (n = 29) and trends in BBA birth 2000–2007 in a large English maternity unit. *MIDIRS Midwifery Digest*, 18, 217–23.

Fullerton, J.T., Navarro, A.M. and Young, S.H. (2007) Outcomes of planned home birth: an integrative review. *Journal of Midwifery and Women's Health*, 52, 323–33.

Gray, M. (2001) *Evidence-based Health Care*. Edinburgh: Churchill Livingstone.

Gyte, G. and Dodwell, M. (2008) Safety of planned home birth: and NCT review of evidence. *MIDIRS Midwifery Digest*, 18, 376–85.

Hodnett, E.D., Downe, S., Edwards, N. and Walsh, D (2005) Home-like versus conventional institutional settings for birth. *Cochrane Database of Systematic Reviews*, Vol. 1, 12 November.

Hodnett, E.D., Gates, S., Hofymer, G.J., Sakala, C. and Weston, J. (2011) Continuous support during childbirth. *Cochrane Database of Systematics Review*, Issue 2.

Hollis Martin, C.J. (2008) Birth planning for midwives and mothers. *British Journal of Midwives*, 16, 583–7.

Holloway, I. and Bluff, R. (1994) 'They know best': women's perceptions of midwifery care during labour. *Midwifery*, 10(5), 157–64.

Homeyard, C. and Gaudion, A. (2008) Safety in maternity services: women's perspectives. *Practising Midwife*, 11(7), 20–3.

House of Commons (1992) *House of Commons Health Committee on Maternity Services Report* (Winterton Report Part 1). London: HMSO.

House of Commons (2003) *House of Commons Health Committee: Choice in Maternity Services*. Ninth Report of Session 2002–3, Vol. 1. HC 796-1. London: The Stationery Office.

House of Commons (2004) *House of Commons Health Committee Provision of Maternity Services*. Fourth Report of Session 2002–3, Vol. 1. HC 464-1. London: The Stationery Office.

van der Hulst, L.M., van Teijlingen, E.R., Bonsel, G.J., Eskes, M. and Bleker, O.P. (2004) Does a pregnant woman's intended place of birth influence her attitudes toward and occurrence of obstetric interventions? *Birth*, 31(1), 28–33.

International Confederation of Midwives (2005) *Definition of the Midwife*. The Hague: International Confederation of Midwives.

Janssen, P.A., Henderson, A.D. and Vedam, S. (2009) The experience of planned home birth: views of the first 500 women. *Birth* 36, 297–304.

Kitzinger, S. (1979) *Birth at Home*. Oxford: Oxford University Press.

Macfarlane, A., McCandlish, R. and Campbell, R. (2000) Choosing between home and hospital delivery (letter). *British Medical Journal*, 320(7237), 798 (http://bmj.bmjjournals.com/cgi/content/full/320/7237/798?; accessed July 2009).

Madden, E. (2005) A birth vision. *Midwives*, 8(2), 68–71.

Morison, S., Hauck, Y., Percival, P. and McMurray, A. (1998) Constructing a homebirth environment through assuming control. *Midwifery*, 14, 233–41.

Morison, S., Hauck, Y., Percival, P. and McMurray, A. (1999) Birthing at home: the resolution of expectations. *Midwifery*, 15(1), 32–9.

NHS Choices: Your Health – Your Choices (http://www.nhs.uk/nhsengland/thenhs/about/pages/nhsstructure.aspx; accessed July 2010)

NHS Choices: Your Health, Your Choice of Birthplace (http://www.nhs.uk/livewell/pregnancy/pages/wheretogivebirth.aspx; accessed July 1010).

National Childbirth Trust (NCT) (http://www.nctpregnancyandbabycare.com/home; accessed July 2010).

National Institute for Health and Clinical Excellence (NICE) (2007) *Intrapartum Care: Care of Healthy Women and Their Babies During Childbirth*. London: RCOG Press (accessible at http://www.nice.org.uk/nicemedia/live/11837/36275/36275.pdf; accessed 5 August 2011).

National Perinatal Epidemiology Unit (2010) Prospective cohort study of planned place of birth (study in progress) (https://www.npeu.ox.ac.uk/birthplace/component-studies/pcsppb; accessed July 2010).

NHS Scotland (2003) Implementing *A Framework for Maternity Services in Scotland*. Edinburgh: Scottish Executive (http://www.scotland.gov.uk/Resource/Doc/47021/0013919.pdf; accessed July 2010).

Nolan, M., Smith, J. and Catling, J. (2009a) Experiences in early labour. 1. Contact with health professionals. *Practising Midwife*, 12(7), 20–5.

Nolan, M., Smith, J. and Catling, J. (2009b) Experiences in early labour. 2. Strategies for coping at home. *Practising Midwife*, 12(8), 36–7.

Northern Region Perinatal Mortality Survey Coordinating Group (1996) Collaborative Survey of Perinatal Loss in Planned and Unplanned Home Birth. *BMJ*, 313, 1306–19.

Nursing and Midwifery Council (2004) *Midwives' Rules and Standards*. M/05/05 January 2005. London: Nursing and Midwifery Council.

Nursing and Midwifery Council (2006) *Midwives and Home Birth*. Circular 08/2006 (http://www.nmc-uk.org/Documents/Circulars/2006%20circulars/NMC%20circular%2008_2006.pdf; accessed July 2006).

Nursing and Midwifery Council (2008) *The Code: Standards of Conduct, Performance and Ethics for Nurses and Midwives*. London: Nursing and Midwifery Council.

Nursing and Midwifery Council (2009a) *Modern Supervision in Action*. London: Nursing and Midwifery Council.

Nursing and Midwifery Council (2009b) *Record Keeping: Guidance for Nurses and Midwives*. London: Nursing and Midwifery Council (http://www.nmc-uk.org; accessed July 2010).

Olsen, O. (1997) Meta-analysis of the safety of home birth. *Birth*, 24(1), 4–13.

Richardson, J. (2009) Supervisory issues: lessons to learn from a home birth. *British Journal of Midwifery*, 17, 710–12.

Royal College of Midwives (2002) *Home Birth Handbook. Vol. 1: Promoting Home Birth*. London: Royal College of Midwives.

Royal College of Midwives (2004) *Position Statement no. 4 – Normal Childbirth*. London: Royal College of Midwives.

Sackett, D.L., Richardson, W.S. and Rosenberg, W. and Haynes, B. (2000) *Evidence-Based Medicine: How to Practice and Teach EBM*, 2nd edn. Edinburgh: Churchill Livingstone.

Singh, D. and Newburn, M. (2000) *Access to Maternity Information and Support: The Needs and Experiences of Pregnant Women and New Mothers*. London: National Childbirth Trust.

Sookhoo, D. (2009) Race and ethnicity. In Squire, C. (ed.) *The Social Context of Birth*, 2nd edn. Abingdon: Radcliffe Publishing.

Stephens, L. (2005) Worrying truth behind home birth figures. *British Journal of Midwifery*, 13, 14–15.

Thomas, P. (1998) *Choosing a Home birth*. London: Association for Improvements in Maternity Services (AIMS).

United Kingdom Parliament (2004) Government Response to House of Commons Health Committee Reports: Fourth Report Session 2002–3, *Provision of Maternity Services*; Eighth Report Session 2002–3, *Inequalities in Access to Maternity Services*; and Ninth Report Session 2002–3, *Choice in Maternity Services* presented to Parliament by the Secretary of State. February 2004. Cm 6140. London: HMSO.

Walsh, D. (2003) Birth as a risky behaviour: reflections on risk management. *MIDIRS Midwifery Digest*, 13, 545–9.

Walsh, D., El-Nemer, A. and Downe, S. (2004) Risk, safety and the study of physiological birth. In Downe, S. (ed.) *Normal Childbirth: The Evidence and the Debate*. Edinburgh: Churchill Livingstone.

Warwick, C. (2004) Setting up a homebirth service. Presentation at Nursing and Midwifery Council Conference, 12 November 2004.

Welsh Assembly Government (2002) Paper 4. *Delivering the Future in Wales: A Framework for Realising the Potential of Nurses, Midwives and Health Visitors in Wales*. Cardiff: Welsh Assembly Government.

Welsh Assembly Government (2005) *National Service Framework for Children, Young People and Maternity Services in Wales*. Cardiff: Welsh Assembly Government.

Wiegers, T., van der Zee, J., Kerrsons, J. and Keirse, M. (2000) Variation in home-birth rates between midwifery practices in the Netherlands. *Midwifery*, 16(2), 96–104.

Wilkins, R. (2000) Poor relations: the paucity of the professional paradigm. In Kirkham, M. (ed.) *The Midwife–Mother Relationship*. London: Macmillan Press.

Chapter 3   **Guidelines to support homebirth**

Bridgid McKeown and Verena Wallace

Introduction

Home birth guidelines aim to facilitate the safe birth of the baby and achieve a satisfactory outcome and experience for the mother. Guidelines are not intended to be prescriptive nor to replace the midwife's clinical judgement, and will change as new or updated evidence emerges.

The principles of developing guidelines and polices are that they should be robust, clear and based on the best available evidence. Cross-reference to other guidelines must be identified. The relevant criteria must be clearly outlined for audit purposes (LSA Midwifery Officers' Forum UK, 2010).

This chapter considers some points that may help when developing or updating homebirth guidelines:

- national guidance;
- local guidelines;
- evidence base;
- information for women;
- roles and responsibilities;
- documentation;
- communication;
- equipment;
- medicines;
- attending a homebirth;
- transfer of care;
- skills for homebirth;
- homebirth and supervision of midwives;
- standards and audit.

National guidance

As members of a regulated profession, midwives are required to work within the Nursing and Midwifery Council's *Midwives' Rules and Standards* (Nursing and Midwifery Council, 2004) and *The Code: Standards of Conduct, Performance and Ethics* (Nursing and Midwifery Council, 2008). It is explicit within the *Midwives' Rules and Standards* that midwives should be competent in caring for women having normal labour and birth and to recognise deviation from the normal, offer evidence-based, accessible information and respect and support women's choice.

Relevant current national documents include:

- *Antenatal Care: Routine Care for the Healthy Pregnant Woman*, Clinical Guideline 62 (National Institute for Health and Clinical Excellence, 2008a);
- *Home Birth Handbook*, Vol. 1 (Royal College of Midwives, 2002);
- *Home Birth Handbook*, Vol. 2 (Royal College of Midwives, 2003);
- *Home Births* (RCOG/RCM, 2007);
- *Induction of Labour*, Clinical Guideline 70 (National Institute for Health and Clinical Excellence, 2008b);
- *Intrapartum Care*, Clinical Guideline 55 (National Institute for Health and Clinical Excellence, 2007);
- *Midwives and Homebirth* (Nursing and Midwifery Council, 2006);
- *Record Keeping: Guidance for Nurses and Midwives* (Nursing and Midwifery Council, 2009a);
- *Routine Postnatal Care of Women and their Babies*, Clinical Guideline 37 (National Institute for Health and Clinical Excellence, 2006);
- *Safer Childbirth* (RCOG *et al.*, 2007);
- *Standards for Medicines Management* (Nursing and Midwifery Council, 2007).

Local guidelines

Homebirth guidelines should clearly define the parameters and scope of the homebirth services. Women, midwives and other agencies need to understand what is and is not included in the provision of the homebirth services. Guidelines should ensure that roles, responsibilities and lines of communication are clear so that appropriate care is provided for women.

Midwives are also required to adhere to regional and local maternity services strategies, which will provide direction and influence how homebirths are managed (Northern Health and Social Care Trust, 2009). Relevant policies and clinical guidelines, for example local clinical risk management policies, should be incorporated.

Other agencies are crucial in the collaborative management of safe homebirth services. Local stakeholders and lay users of the services, such as the National Childbirth Trust (NCT) or Maternity Services Liaison Committee (MSLC), should be identified and involved in the development of local guidelines. Midwives, working with the multidisciplinary team, should discuss service interfaces and agree protocols for referral and transfer of care.

The NCT highlighted the need for robust transfer arrangements between the ambulance service and the medical and midwifery staff receiving the women at the hospital (Gyte and Dodwell, 2007). The regional ambulance service and paramedics should be involved in developing a service level agreement and joint protocols for emergency transfer from home to hospital should the need arise.

General practitioners' (GPs') knowledge of an individual woman's medical history is crucial, and guidelines should outline how this information will be communicated to midwives providing home birth services. The Royal College of Obstetricians and Gynaecologists (RCOG, in its response to the King's Fund discussion paper on 'The role of GPs in maternity care – what does the future hold?', welcomed more effective multidisciplinary team working between GPs, midwives and obstetricians (RCOG, 2010). GPs should be encouraged to provide comprehensive information about the woman's medical, social and mental health history (NHS Quality Improvement Scotland, 2004), using the most effective communication method available to them and their midwifery colleagues.

Evidence base

In 2009, in the four countries of the UK, the average percentage of homebirths ranged from 0.37 per cent in Northern Ireland to 3.83 per cent in Wales (BirthChoiceUK website). Implicit in government policy in all four countries is the promotion of choice for women in relation to their pregnancy care and place of birth (Department of Health, 2007; Scottish Government, 2011). This includes being offered the choice of planning a birth at home.

When developing guidelines, the first step should be a literature search to inform both the guidelines and accompanying information for women. Where national guidance from sources such as the National Institute for Health and Clinical Excellence (NICE) has been adopted, this should be reflected in local guidelines.

NICE advocates offering women choice when planning the place of birth and acknowledges that giving birth is generally very safe for both the woman and her baby (National Institute for Health and Clinical Excellence, 2007). It suggests that women who plan to give birth at home or in a midwife-led unit (MLU) have a higher likelihood of a normal birth, with less intervention. This agrees with previous work by Janssen and colleagues (2002), Ackermann-Liebrich and colleagues (1996) and Woodcock and colleagues (1990, 1994). However, NICE (National Institute for Health and Clinical Excellence, 2007) states 'we do not have enough information about the possible risks to either the woman or the baby relating to planned place of birth'.

In addition, NICE (National Institute for Health and Clinical Excellence, 2007) states that 'if something does go unexpectedly seriously wrong during labour at home or in a midwifery led unit, the outcome for the woman and baby could be worse than if they were in the obstetric unit with access to specialised care'. NICE suggests that women with pre-existing medical conditions or previous complicated births should be advised to give birth in an obstetric unit.

A Cochrane review reported by Olsen and Jewell (1998) found no strong evidence against benefits and safety of planned homebirth compared with hospital birth for low-risk women. It was noted that the increase in planned hospital births for low-risk women that took place in many countries during the twentieth century was not supported by good evidence. Planned hospital birth may even increase unnecessary interventions and complications without any benefit for low-risk women Nine years later, the NCT reviewed the available evidence on the safety of planned homebirths compared with planned hospital births (Gyte and Dodwell, 2007). It also evaluated the safety of women at risk of complications and reviewed perinatal mortality outcomes, that is, babies dying during labour or shortly after birth. It concluded that there was no evidence to suggest that hospital birth is safer than homebirth for low-risk women and called for the needs of women to be met irrespective of the place of birth.

Further publications on the safety of homebirths include those by Mori and colleagues (2008), de Jonge and colleagues (2009) and Wax and colleagues (2010), which have generated much debate. Wax and colleagues (2010) suggest that childbirth in the UK remains very safe. Although transfers and unplanned homebirths appear to carry higher risk for the baby (Mori *et al.*, 2008; Wax *et al.*, 2010), de Jonge and colleagues (2009) suggest that planned homebirth for low-risk women does not increase the risks of perinatal mortality and severe morbidity in the newborn. There are many good sources of debate about the articles such as in the NHS Knowledge Service on the NHS Choices website.

The National Perinatal Epidemiology Unit (NPEU), University of Oxford, has been commissioned to research how the current provision of maternity services in England affects safety, quality of care and women's childbirth experiences. The 'Birthplace' study, which commenced in September 2006 (National Perinatal Epidemiology Unit, 2010), will also evaluate costs associated with systems of care and processes between services and is due to report in September 2011.

Information for women

The development of information for women about local homebirth services is inextricably linked to clinical guidelines. Evidence-based information for women about homebirths should be up to date and the potential benefits, known risks and uncertainties should be discussed when planning place of birth.

It was recommended in *Safer Childbirth* (RCOG *et al.*, 2007) that women should be helped to make an informed choice about where they wish to give birth. Rule 2 of the *Midwives' Rules and Standards* advises the midwife to 'discuss matters fully' and make sure that the woman and her baby are the 'primary focus of her practice' (Nursing and Midwifery Council, 2004). Any written information should include signposting to reputable sources such as the Nursing and Midwifery Council (NMC), NICE, the Royal College of Midwives (RCM), RCOG and Quality Improvement Scotland (QIS).

RCOG/RCM (2007) advocates offering the option of a homebirth to all women with uncomplicated pregnancies, stating that homebirths are safe for many women and that, if given true choices, around 8–10 per cent of women would opt for a homebirth. However, as homebirth is not the best option for all women, evidence-based guidance and information for women will help the woman and her midwife to consider all the options for place of birth. Discussions should take into consideration individual circumstance, wishes, knowledge and known and potential risks.

Women may plan to give birth at home for a variety of reasons. Some express utmost confidence in their ability to birth safely at home regardless of any identified risk factors. Some may have had a previous negative experience in hospital. Others may feel that giving birth at home will provide a more spiritual, family-centred experience. Regardless of the reasons why women choose to give birth at home, midwives can empower and assist them to have an experience that is as emotionally satisfying and as safe as possible.

RCOG *et al.* (2007) recommend that written information regarding choices about the place of birth should be available to all women. Sharing and discussing local homebirth guidelines with women who choose this option of care will help clarify what is available, what is not and how services are organised. The provision of evidence-based information and taking time to discuss the practicalities and implications of homebirths assists the woman to make her choice.

As well as available literature, websites such as the NCT (http://www.nct.org.uk/home), NHS Choices (http://www.nhs.uk/Pages/HomePage.aspx) and NICE (http://www.nice.org.uk/) provide useful information to help parents make decisions about homebirths. Working together to identify potential risks and challenges in the context of the woman's individual circumstances is good practice.

In preparation for the homebirth women will seek relevant information from various sources. Some women may choose to access information via friends or relatives or use the internet but they all will require local information about how the homebirth will be facilitated. Guidelines should emphasise the requirement for antenatal discussion time between the women and her midwife about birth choices. Discussions may take place during antenatal appointments, group education classes or one-to-one sessions. Topics may include active birth advice, birth story dialogues and pain management. Relevant evidence-based information such as the timing and possible methods for induction of labour should also be included (National Institute for Health and Clinical Excellence, 2008b). Information may be made available from the midwife or reiterated using leaflets, websites or DVDs.

Women should be informed how to recognise the signs of normal early labour and be aware of when and how to call the midwife, particularly in an emergency (Appendix 3.1). Appendix 3.2 provides advice for the woman or her birth partner on what to say if involved in calling an emergency ambulance during the home birth as well as a situation, background, assessment and recommendation (SBAR) tool for completion by the midwife prior to transfer.

Roles and responsibilities

Essentially the role of the midwife providing a homebirth service is to:

- work in partnership with the woman, partner, family and the other professionals involved in the woman's care;
- provide evidence-based care throughout the woman's pregnancy and birth and in the postnatal period;
- support the woman's individual needs and expectations, whilst ensuring safety for the woman and her baby;
- provide comprehensive evidence-based information enabling the woman to make informed decisions.

Birth in any setting is an emotional occasion, and mothers and fathers will remember their birth stories for the rest of their lives. Midwives are privileged to be part of such a joyous event in the woman's own home and, like all significant events, homebirths are most successful when properly planned and prepared for.

Planning

Planning a homebirth is an important life choice, and so not all women will have made a firm decision by their first antenatal appointment. As advocated by NICE (National Institute for Health and Clinical Excellence, 2008a), lower-risk women now have fewer appointments, which may limit opportunities to discuss any issues or concerns. Homebirth should be mentioned as a choice at the beginning of the woman's engagement with maternity services and, if the woman expresses interest in a homebirth, planning can start early in her pregnancy (Royal College of Midwives, 2002). Midwives should have a visible place in a community setting where women can choose to access them as the first point of contact. The midwife is the lead professional for homebirths and will coordinate women's care through pregnancy and until the end of the postnatal period (Midwifery 2020, 2010).

It is expected that midwives will offer the same level of evidence-based antenatal care and screening regardless of the planned location for the birth. An additional antenatal clinic appointment or an early home visit can be arranged to facilitate questions and decision-making. This also provides an opportunity for the midwife to get to know the woman and gain greater insight into her needs and wishes for birth.

Assessment

Conflict sometimes arises over whether or not the woman is making a choice that places her or her unborn child at risk (Walsh *et al.*, 2004). In the absence of strong evidence on assessment for choosing place of birth, NICE has produced guidance to use when considering the relative risk associated with place of birth so that the mother can make the choice with the best information available (National Institute for Health and Clinical Excellence, 2007).

RCOG/RCM (2007) acknowledged there were no known risk assessment tools which can effectively predict outcomes for pregnancy and labour. Lewis (2007) called for a formal risk assessment tool to maintain a consistent approach to recognising and managing risks. A risk assessment tool provides an invaluable form of documentation for recording discussions about identified and potential risks and for planning alternative options for care. Service providers should have locally agreed risk assessment tools as an appendix in their guidelines.

The best approach to assessment is to commence it at 'booking' and to continuously assess risk throughout the woman's pregnancy, labour and postnatal period. The booking history should include a review of the referral letter and use of local computerised maternity information systems such as the Northern Ireland Maternity Services Information System (NIMATS), the Scottish Women Hand-Held Maternity Record (SWHHMR) or Euroking (used in other parts of the UK). A printed copy of the booking report should be inserted in the maternity hand-held record (MHHR). Taking a sound history will generate discussion about any identified challenges and prompt discussions about how they can be managed. For example, the woman will need to reassess the choices she has made if the midwife identifies that a planned birth in an obstetric unit is more appropriate.

Women have a right to make their own decisions; the midwife should be straightforward and clear in the discussions about identified risks or challenges and potential circumstances in which transfer of care to a consultant obstetrician would be recommended. The midwife must be realistic about what the midwives can or cannot do in the home setting. Advice should be specific rather than non-directional, and women who have known risk factors which indicate a poor obstetric outcome should be offered a consultant obstetrician appointment. Women deemed to be at higher risk should be actively encouraged to give birth in a consultant-led maternity unit.

Having made the options clear, the midwife should facilitate and respect the woman's decisions (provided she has the capacity to make that decision). It is important for the midwife to uphold women's rights to be fully involved in decisions about their care and to respect and support a woman's right to accept or decline treatment and care. The midwife should document the options, benefits, risks and any discussions and advice she has given to the woman in the hand-held maternity notes.

Documentation

Guidelines should list, in appendices, all the necessary documentation for a homebirth. Examples are:

- Notification of Request for Homebirth (local);
- Notification of Birth;
- Notification of Completed Homebirth (local);
- Personal Child Health Record (PCHR).

In some areas the midwife's method for informing his or her midwifery manager of a planned homebirth is to use a 'Notification of Request for Homebirth' proforma. A copy is inserted in the woman's hand-held notes (Appendix 3.3).

Following the birth, a midwife present at the birth will complete the 'Notification of Birth' form to notify the Registrar and to ensure entry onto local child health systems. The NHS number (UK) or Health and Care Number (Northern Ireland) will be initiated and the PCHR given to the mother. The midwife should explain the processes for registering the birth at the local council office and with the GP.

The manager should be informed verbally or in writing of the outcome of the homebirth. Some trusts use a Notification of Completed Homebirth proforma (Appendix 3.4), which can subsequently facilitate local audits.

Conversely, audits also need to consider circumstances in which transfer was indicated but did not occur, for example if the woman refused transfer and remained at home. Audits of homebirths should be carried out regularly and inform the Trust and supervisor of midwives' clinical governance networks.

It is important to record the information and advice given, recommended actions and any decisions made in the woman's notes. All documentation should meet the standards in *Record Keeping: Guidance for Nurses and Midwives* (Nursing and Midwifery Council, 2009a).

Communication

A care pathway can be useful communication tool to include in guidelines as an appendix to assist midwives to plan woman-focused care and ensure that clinical activities are coordinated at the appropriate times. The woman has the choice whether to accept all or some of the care options. Care pathways are not rigid documents, and midwives should use their own professional judgement in response to the woman's individual needs or wishes. The care pathway should be reviewed at each appointment and deviations from the pathway and the woman's decisions should be recorded on the MHHR. A pathway may be useful for guiding midwives who are inexperienced in managing homebirths, that is, in areas where low homebirth rates result in limited opportunities to gain experience of birth in a community setting.

Most homebirth care pathways will recommend an antenatal home visit at about 36 weeks to discuss the woman's hopes and concerns and clarify the midwife's role at the homebirth. This is a good opportunity to confirm that basic requirements and telephone access are available. The RCM (Royal College of Midwives, 2003) provides detailed guidance on preparation for homebirth, including the consideration of issues such as the birthing area having ready access to hot and cold water, toilet facilities, space to mobilise, adequate heating and good light.

Prior to the birth, in the interests of good communication and teamworking, the midwife should communicate the woman's name, address, telephone number, parity, expected date of delivery (EDD), any identified risk factors, the on-call rota and midwife bleep or mobile telephone contact details to:

- the woman and her birth partner;
- midwives on the on-call rota;
- local maternity unit – delivery suite midwife in charge (and/or hospital switchboard);
- community midwifery team leader;
- supervisor of midwives on-call.

It is a midwife's duty to identify the perceived benefits and possible risks associated with different options within the context of the woman's individual circumstances. A woman can make the choice for a particular place of birth at any stage in pregnancy. The presence or absence of risk may change during pregnancy and labour and the midwife must continuously assess the advice she gives to the woman. The midwife must take care to pre-plan to mitigate identified risks through her approach to care, utilise knowledge of local help and emergency systems and communicate effectively with colleagues and the woman and her family.

Use of technology

Access to internet-based maps can help to make sure that everyone knows exactly where the woman's home is and how to get to it. Satellite navigation systems may be useful particularly in rural areas for those midwives with access, as are mobile phones and web-based evidence information targeted at pregnant women.

In areas with little or no mobile phone coverage, suitable arrangements should be made in advance of the birth for land line telephone access.

Birth plan

A written birth plan (Appendix 3.5) is a useful communication tool for clarifying the woman's intentions for pain management and for outlining her arrangements for other children and pets during her birth. Although not every woman will use a birth plan, the majority will wish to discuss arrangements and options for care during labour. Most women will want their birth partner present during labour, and some like to hire a doula for additional emotional and practical support. Most hand held notes include a birth plan which may be enough, but if required an outline birth plan for homebirth can be included as an appendix in the guideline and a completed version inserted into the woman's MHHR prior to labour.

After the birth

The midwife should provide leaflets and discuss information during the ante-natal period such as:

- anti-D (National for Health and Clinical Excellence, 2008c);
- examination of the newborn;
- neonatal blood spot test;

- neonatal hearing test;
- tuberculosis screening and vaccination.

After the baby's birth, follow-up postnatal care at home is arranged according to the mother's and baby's needs and wishes and at the midwife's discretion. The routine newborn baby examination and screening tests should be offered and arranged with the mother's consent.

Equipment

Appendix 3.6 shows a sample equipment list for homebirth which can be adapted. Guidance should confirm that each on-call midwife is responsible for ensuring that the necessary equipment is available, well maintained, serviced in accordance with manufacturer's instructions and tested before each homebirth. The RCM (Royal College of Midwives, 2003) recommends using a small, easily cleaned, wheeled suitcase containing only essential equipment. Resuscitation equipment should be kept in a separate bag that is easy to access in an emergency.

In some areas in the UK, midwives bring the equipment when called to the birth. Alternatively, the equipment may be left at the home during the 36th week and stored in a cool dry place away from direct heat, preferably in a secure room. Arrangements for disposal of waste products, 'sharps' boxes and the placenta after the homebirth should be made clear in the local guidance (usually at the local hospital). Disposable instruments are favoured in the interests of infection control, and should be disposed of in a 'sharps' box. If the woman wishes to keep her own placenta this should be documented in the notes. Otherwise, the placenta should be dealt with according to local health and safety and infection control policies that are made explicit in the local homebirth guidance. The equipment must be returned, checked, cleaned and restocked in preparation for the next homebirth.

Medicines

It is good practice for the guidelines to include a list of necessary medications and written advice on the safe storage of medicines, medical gases and equipment. The woman should be advised to arrange any GP prescriptions and to be aware of the contraindications and known side-effects documented in the medication 'patient information' leaflets. All medications administered should be recorded in the MHHR and in accordance with NMC standards for medicines management (Nursing and Midwifery Council, 2007).

Guidelines should be clear about pain management options available to women at home. Anecdotal evidence suggests that opioid use is decreasing in homebirths. It should be noted that some trusts are implementing a minimum postadministration observation period of five hours as opioids may cause short-term respiratory depression and drowsiness. These side-effects may last for several days in the baby and may interfere with breast-feeding (National Institute for Health and Clinical Excellence, 2007). Changes in practice may limit pain relief options at home, and this must be identified in information for women and well as in guidance for midwives.

Midwife supply order

Historically, if there were difficulties with the GP prescribing controlled drugs for a homebirth, a midwife supply order (MSO) was used. Although uncommon now, to obtain a midwife supply order supervisors of midwives should contact their local supervising authority midwifery officer (LSAMO).

Midwives' exemptions

Under legislation, registered midwives may supply and administer (but not prescribe), on their own initiative, any of the medicines identified under midwives' exemptions, provided this is done in the course of their professional midwifery practice. For the medicines specified under the midwives' exemptions they do not require a prescription, patient-specific direction (PSD) from a medical practitioner or a patient group direction (PGD), provided the conditions attached to the midwives' exemptions are met. It should be noted that any medicine not included under the midwives' exemptions requires a PGD, prescription or a PSD (Nursing and Midwifery Council, 2011).

Midwives are reminded that, in addition to the prescription-only medicines (PoM) listed in Annexe 1 of *Changes to Midwives' Exemptions* (Nursing and Midwifery Council, 2011), they have access to all pharmacy (P) and general sales list (GSL) medicines provided such access is necessary in the course of their professional practice.

When supplying or administering medicines under midwives' exemptions, midwives must have received the appropriate training in therapeutic use, dosage, side-effects, precautions, contraindications and methods of administration and must ensure that their practice is evidence based (Nursing and Midwifery Council, 2011).

If midwives are unclear about midwives' exemptions and homebirth medicines supply and administration, they must check with their supervisor of midwives.

Medical gases

Local arrangements for obtaining medical gases should be explicit in the homebirth guidelines and explained to the woman and her family. Historically in some areas GPs prescribed medical gases (oxygen and Entonox) which the community pharmacist delivered to the woman's home. In other areas, midwives have arranged for transport of gas cylinders from the hospital or community pharmacy to the home. In the past if midwives transported medical gases in their cars, suitable motor insurance had to be in place, but this practice is now rare and not recommended.

Medical gas cylinders should be handled carefully and stored safely in accordance with supplier's guidelines.

Attending a homebirth

The on-call system depends on the local service delivery model and should be outlined in the guidance. Case load and team midwives usually provide a rolling on-call arrangement covering 24 hours a day, seven days a week. In areas where traditional community midwifery models operate, the rota should be prepared and agreed with colleagues before 37 weeks. All midwives involved should arrange to visit the woman at home to introduce themselves, discuss the birth plan, check directions, clarify predicted response times and check mobile phone coverage.

The 'first on call' midwife should be called when the woman feels she is in established labour or if the membranes rupture. As the length of the first stage of labour may vary, the first midwife will assess the stage of labour, offer support and agree a plan of action. If the woman does not appear to be in established labour, the plan may be for the midwife to leave to organise other duties, whilst maintaining contact and to return later. Once established labour is confirmed, the first midwife will notify the second midwife on-call and the named support delivery suite. Following the birth the midwife who is in attendance should inform all relevant services of the outcome of the homebirth, that is, delivery suite, community midwifery manager/team leader, supervisor of midwives on call.

Transfer of care

Should the woman reconsider her homebirth plan, request an epidural or develop risk factors, then care should be transferred to the appropriate maternity unit. This must be clearly identified as a transfer of care and documented in the women's MHHR. Where trusts have a form specifically for transfer of care between specialties or between midwife and consultant-led care, and where available, this form should be used (see Appendix 3.2).

Although the study was carried out some time ago, it is useful for women to be aware of the National Birthday Trust Report, a comprehensive study of homebirths, which reported that 40 per cent of primigravid women are transferred to hospital in labour compared with 10 per cent of multigravid women. The 'single largest reason for transfer was slow progress in labour' (Chamberlain *et al.*, 1997). More recently, the National Collaborating Centre for Women's and Children's Health study suggested that, on average, around 14 per cent of women who have chosen a homebirth will be transferred – although the figure is significantly higher for first-time mothers and significantly lower for parous women (Mori *et al.*, 2008).

Emergency transfer during labour

During the antenatal period the midwife has a responsibility to clearly discuss the possible impact on the well-being of the woman and baby should adverse events occur during labour. Discussions should include:

- the perceived risks, reason for transfer and likelihood of transfer;
- what can be done and any limitations;
- mode of transport, for example 999 'blue light' ambulance;
- the name of the emergency back-up hospital;
- the estimated transfer time to hospital, which may vary according to local circumstances, for example prevailing weather conditions, roadworks.

During labour there should be ongoing assessments, and in the event of an obstetric emergency agreed local procedures and guidelines should be followed. Reasons for the transfer should be explained and arrangements made to transfer the woman and baby (if already born) to the named hospital. If both midwives are busy, a family member can be instructed to call a 'blue light' emergency '999' ambulance with a paramedic support for 'an obstetric emergency at a homebirth'. The caller must give the woman's name, address and telephone number and clear directions if the home is difficult to locate (Appendix 3.2).

Emergency care must be continued until handover to the paramedic or obstetric staff as appropriate. Effective communication includes a full verbal and written report on the relevant history, reason for transfer, perceived risks, observations, actions taken and medication history. The midwife should accompany the woman in the ambulance and hand over to the senior hospital midwife or obstetrician. The obstetrician accepting the case should make a full assessment and plan of management. Full documentation of observations, reason for transfer and actions taken should be recorded and the notes should be transferred with the woman. An example of an SBAR (situation, background, assessment, recommendations) tool is available in Appendix 3.2 and if used should be filed in the woman's notes.

Any baby who gives the midwife cause for concern should be transferred immediately to a hospital with appropriate neonatal services. If necessary, emergency neonatal resuscitation should be commenced. The midwife should accompany the baby in the ambulance and hand over to the senior hospital midwife, neonatologist or paediatrician. The person accepting the case should make a full assessment and plan of management. Full documentation of observations, reason for transfer and actions taken should be recorded and the notes should be transferred with the baby.

'Flying squads'

The RCM and RCOG no longer support the use of flying squads. Therefore, in the event of an emergency, transfer to the nearest obstetric unit by paramedic ambulance is considered best practice (RCOG/RCM, 2007).

Other agencies are crucial in the collaborative management of homebirth services, particularly the regional ambulance service. Paramedics should be involved in developing a service level agreement and joint protocols for transfers from homebirths so that midwives and paramedics are clear about each other's skills and responsibilities.

Rare events

In the rare, sad event of a stillbirth, neonatal death or maternal death occurring at home, the emergency services will be called and support and guidance sought immediately from the on-call supervisor of midwives and the midwifery manager. Midwives should ensure that they are familiar with their local supervision of midwives guidelines, which will signpost how to proceed with continued care provision and the required investigations in these exceptional circumstances.

Skills for homebirths

There are a range of essential skills common to all midwifery practice regardless of the place of birth. All midwives need to:

- be knowledgeable, up to date and aware of current local and national guidelines;
- ensure that women receive evidence-based information in order to facilitate informed choice;
- be competent in observing, assessing and understanding the physiological changes associated with pregnancy and childbirth;
- consider the woman's emotional and psychological needs and coping strategies;
- understand the principles of risk assessment and be able to recognise and respond to deviations from the norm and make appropriate referrals;
- be able to discuss challenges and suitable options with the woman and partner in a sensitive, objective manner;
- employ emergency care skills when required;
- have good multidisciplinary teamworking skills;
- have good record-keeping skills;
- use information technology appropriately for care.

A midwife must possess the knowledge, skills and abilities for lawful, safe and effective practice on the midwife's own responsibility and accountability. This will include competent care throughout the antenatal, intrapartum and postnatal periods (Nursing and Midwifery Council, 2009b).

As a member of a self-regulating profession, each midwife is responsible for maintaining and developing his or her own skills and competence. According to *The Code: Standards of Conduct, Performance and Ethics for Nurses and Midwives* (Nursing and Midwifery Council, 2008), midwives must:

- recognise and work within the limits of their competence;
- keep their knowledge and skills up to date throughout their working life;
- take part in appropriate learning and practice activities that maintain and develop their competence and performance.

Rule 2 specifies that 'key midwifery skills include anticipation and forward planning' (Nursing and Midwifery Council, 2004). The timely recognition, referral and treatment of any woman who is developing a critical illness during or after pregnancy is of critical importance (CMACE 2011, p. 11). Keen observation of early abnormal physical signs and symptoms should alert the midwife to the possibility of serious illness warranting immediate medical referral.

Rule 6 (Nursing and Midwifery Council, 2004) outlines the midwife's responsibilities for providing care within her sphere of practice. However, although recognised as expert in normal childbirth at the point of registration, many midwives develop their childbirth skills within a hospital environment, and some have little or no experience of homebirths pre or post registration. Pre-registration student midwives should be encouraged and facilitated to avail themselves of every opportunity to gain experience in attending homebirths.

Rule 6 (Nursing and Midwifery Council, 2004) directs midwives on actions to take: 'in an emergency . . . a practising midwife shall call such qualified health professional as may reasonably be expected to have the necessary skills and experience to assist her in the provision of care'. However, in the absence of medical assistance the midwife should be 'appropriately prepared and clinically up-to-date to ensure that you can carry out effectively, emergency procedures such as resuscitation, for the woman or baby' (Nursing and Midwifery Council, 2004).

The EU Second Midwifery Directive 80/155/EEC, Article 4, section referring to activities of the midwife, includes resuscitation of the woman or baby, and in urgent or emergency circumstances breech delivery, manual removal of placenta and manual examination of the uterus (Nursing and Midwifery Council, 2004, p. 37).

In 2009, a multidisciplinary panel of experienced maternity services staff considered the skills required for a homebirth as part of their case–control retrospective study (CMACE, 2009). The group considered the key skills that midwives should be expected to have to:

- intravenous cannulation;
- suturing the perineum;
- resuscitation of the baby;
- resuscitation of the mother;
- dealing with obstetric emergencies.

Acquiring these skills, if midwives have not been regularly working in an integrated service or in a birthing environment, is a challenge. There are several ways of updating skills for obstetric emergencies.

Many providers commission the Advanced Life Support in Obstetrics (ALSO) or Practical Obstetric Multiprofessional Training (PROMPT) courses for their staff. These courses prepare individuals to deal with emergencies. Both PROMPT and ALSO are multidisciplinary and can take homebirth scenarios into consideration.

NICE (National Institute for Health and Clinical Excellence, 2007) acknowledges that lack of confidence and competence can be a barrier to successful homebirths. Women will know intuitively if a midwife is not comfortable with planning or attending a home birth and this may be particularly pertinent if a 'higher' risk woman chooses to remain at home and the midwife anticipates difficulties at the birth. Forward planning by taking expert advice and reviewing all known risk factors with a constructive attitude will help, and midwives in this position may need to reflect with their supervisor of midwives on their previous experience, values, beliefs and competencies. If a midwife feels she does not have the level of expertise required for homebirth, she must take steps to increase her skills and knowledge by consulting her manager and supervisor of midwives.

Continuing professional development

Midwives undertaking homebirths must be able to manage obstetric and neo-natal emergencies, and should practise these skills regularly (RCOG/RCM, 2007). Although the employer is responsible for staff having the appropriate skills and knowledge levels and should ensure that midwives are fit for their job (Nursing and Midwifery Council, 2010a), the midwife should seek help from her manager or supervisor of midwives to identify additional skills specific to providing care in the home setting and to gain support to update her knowledge and skills.

There are various ways to gain the necessary experience including:

- arranging to work in the maternity unit on a regular or rotational basis to update normal birth and emergency procedure skills;
- using peer support and network with experienced midwifery and medical staff within a maternity unit and externally;
- arranging to shadow or be supervised by an experienced colleague at a homebirth;
- attending team reviews and debriefings to facilitate learning from incidents about positive as well as negative aspects of care.

In the case that a midwife does not have the required experience to meet a woman's specific needs or requests, the midwife must not provide care that she is not competent to give. However, it is not acceptable to refuse to care for a woman on this basis and take no further action (Nursing and Midwifery Council, 2006). The midwife should:

- act as an advocate for the woman, helping her access support, information and appropriate care;
- refer the care of this woman to a colleague with the necessary skills set and take steps to update to become competent herself;
- seek the support of her manager and supervisor of midwives.

Providers (Trusts or Boards) should encourage staff to take time out to practise skills and drills, during which they gain from peer support and constructive criticism in a safe environment. One simple but effective exercise is to empty the resuscitation equipment bag, reflect on the value of each piece of equipment and practise emergency drills using real-life scenarios (Royal College of Midwives, 2003). In the Ulster Maternity Unit in Belfast, the in-house obstetric emergencies training uses real time, real settings, real teams and a video camera to improve the training and learning around obstetric emergency (Madden and McMechan, 2010). The South Eastern Trust has also started joint updating with midwives and paramedics on obstetric emergencies, resuscitation and transfer arrangements from a MLU setting.

Brown and colleagues (2010) take this a step further in Bradford by providing a community skills day in a real-life home environment which brings together community midwives with different levels of experience from across the city. They share experiences and learn together, developing ways of supporting women birthing their babies at home and practise management of emergencies which may unexpectedly develop.

However the updating is organised, basic, immediate and advanced life support training needs must first be identified, then the updating facilitated and evaluated. RCOG/RCM (2007) recognises that commissioning advanced courses may require adequate funding. Managers should keep up-to-date training registers to ensure that all staff participate regularly and are competent in managing births and emergencies at home.

Homebirth and supervision of midwives

> Supervision is a statutory responsibility which provides a mechanism for support and guidance to every midwife practising in the United Kingdom. The purpose of supervision of midwives is to protect women and babies by actively promoting a safe standard of midwifery practice.
>
> (Local Supervising Authority (LSA) Midwifery Officers Forum (UK)/NMC, 2009)

The NMC (Nursing and Midwifery Council, 2006) recognises that there are times when it can be challenging for a midwife to balance the regulatory requirements, comply with local guidelines and support all women who choose to have a homebirth.

> If a midwife is concerned that a woman is making a choice that is not readily available, she should make her concerns known to the manager

of the service in the first instance. If this is not successful in resolving the problem, the midwife should make this known to her supervisor of midwives who has a duty to advise and support her in upholding safety and supporting a woman's choice.

(Nursing and Midwifery Council, 2006)

However, although the guidance is clear about a woman's right to request a homebirth (National Institute for Health and Clinical Excellence, 2007), at present there is no statutory requirement for Trusts to facilitate homebirths. Women who have planned a homebirth find it frustrating and disappointing if they are later informed that the service cannot be accommodated, for example because of staffing problems. Many Trusts recommend that two midwives should be present for the birth, and this can have resource implications. According to RCOG/RCM (2007), withdrawing homebirth services at a late stage is unacceptable.

Every NHS organisation that offers a homebirth service should have clear guidance and contingency plans in place for the escalation of any concerns if it proves difficult to facilitate a homebirth [this should include alerting the supervisors of midwives and the local supervising authority (LSA)].

In order to provide comprehensive care for women who request a homebirth, a supervisor should be involved in developing, reviewing and auditing the use of each NHS Trust's locally agreed policies, guidelines and information leaflets. Supervisors should ensure that local guidance facilitates informed choices for women as recommended in NMC circular on homebirth (Nursing and Midwifery Council, 2006). Homebirths should be discussed proactively as a regular agenda item at supervisors' meetings so that all supervisors are aware of the issues, rates and the outcomes of homebirths.

Safety and/or capacity issues should be discussed at supervisors' meetings in advance or with the on-call supervisor and the head of midwifery in urgent situations. Supervisory teams should ensure that women are informed that they can access a supervisor of midwives or the LSA midwifery officer for support and advice (Nursing and Midwifery Council, 2010b).

If there are perceived significant risks, the midwife should seek further advice from her manager and supervisor of midwives. If the woman continues to plan to give birth at home against professional advice, the manager or supervisor of midwives and the midwife should arrange to meet the woman to discuss options for care. Alternative options may include the local obstetrician-led maternity unit, birth centre, midwife-led unit, or 'DOMINO' support. 'DOMINO' refers to the *dom*iciliary *in* and *out* model whereby the woman plans to give birth in a hospital setting supported by a 'domiciliary' or community midwife. DOMINO may be a suitable option for women who are considered to be at higher risk of complications but who wish to retain continued support from a local midwife:

> if a woman rejects your [the midwife's] advice, you [the midwife] should seek further guidance from your supervisor of midwives to ensure that all possibilities have been explored and that the outcome is appropriately documented . . . You [the midwife] must continue to give the best care you possibly can.
>
> (Woodcock *et al.*, 1990)

If a mutually acceptable option cannot be agreed, the midwife should continue to give the best possible care, seeking support and advice from other members of the health care team, including the supervisor of midwives, as necessary.

For all women it is good practice for the midwife and the woman to agree a plan of care and the action that will be taken should problems arise. If the woman (and/or baby) has complex care needs then a tripartite meeting between the woman, midwife and manager or supervisor of midwives may be helpful in drawing up and documenting a plan of care. Advice and guidance should be sought from the multiprofessional team where appropriate, and further meetings arranged if necessary. Discussions and decisions should be documented in the MHHR. The supervisor of midwives can also obtain further advice from the LSA midwifery officer.

If it becomes apparent to an LSA that midwives are experiencing difficulties in meeting the standards set within *The Code* or *Midwives' Rules*, then the LSA midwifery office should be advising and guiding commissioners and providers to ensure appropriate systems are in place.

The NMC (Nursing and Midwifery Council, 2006) reports that the most common difficulties/barriers identified by women around accessing a homebirth are:

- perceived conflict between risk and a woman's choice;
- confidence and competence of midwives;
- resources.

If a woman has formally indicated that she wants to give birth at home and has booked a homebirth, then she will expect to have a midwife available for a homebirth when she goes into labour. *The Code* (Nursing and Midwifery Council, 2008) confirms that individuals have the right to expect their health care professional to act 'as an advocate for those in your care, helping them to access relevant health and social care, information and support'.

Midwives have a professional responsibility to keep up to date in order to facilitate a woman's choice and to promote a safe standard of midwifery practice. Concurrently, commissioners and service providers need to have the following in place to support midwives to deliver of a range of care options:

- local evidence-based guidelines;
- appropriate and accessible services;
- resources and capacity to respond to a range of maternity care options;
- up-to-date information on place of birth for women and their families.

The *Midwives' Rules and Standards* (Nursing and Midwifery Council, 2004) and *The Code* (Nursing and Midwifery Council, 2008) protect women and at the same time protect midwives by providing a sound framework for their practice.

Standards and audit

Implementation of the homebirth guidelines should be monitored and standards audited. The rationale is that 'care in labour should be aimed towards achieving the best possible outcome for the woman and baby. All maternity services should have in place approved documentation to support the staff who care for women in labour' (NHS Litigation Authority, 2010). An example is in the key performance indicators (KPIs) identified in the Clinical Negligence Scheme for Trusts (CNST) Maternity standards 2010/11, standard 2, criterion 1, 'care of women in labour': 'the maternity service has an approved system for improving care and learning lessons relating to the care of women in labour that is implemented and monitored' (NHS Litigation Authority, 2010).

The context for audit includes:

- frequency of the audit;
- coordination and responsibility for the audit;
- reporting arrangements;
- acting on the recommendations;
- changes in practice and lessons learned;
- links to clinical governance including supervision of midwives;
- feedback to stakeholders.

Conclusion

Effective, safe maternity systems facilitate a range of choices for pregnant women including homebirth. Homebirth guidelines provide information which will help midwives facilitate the safe birth of the baby and achieve a satisfactory outcome and experience for the mother and her family.

As discussed in this chapter, the key points for developing local guidelines include identification of stakeholders and awareness of national guidelines, policies and evidence-based care and local policies and information. The guidelines need to outline the midwife's role and responsibilities and the essential skills and resources required at homebirths. Guidelines should not replace the midwife's clinical judgement and they should assist with assessment, advance planning and dealing with emergencies. Barriers to the provision of homebirths and the key role of commissioners and service providers need to be explored. Supervisors of midwives have an important role to play in the development of the guidelines and in providing advice and support to midwives and women in complex cases.

Midwives have a responsibility to ensure that a woman considering a homebirth receives evidence-based care that is based on a partnership approach which respects the individuality of the woman and her family. Women have the right to make their own decisions on these issues (if they are competent to do so) using evidence-based information, and midwives have a duty of care to respect a woman's choice.

References

Ackermann-Liebrich, U., Voegeli, T., Gunter-Witt, K., Kunz, I., Zullig, M., Schindler, C., Maurer, M. and the Zurich Study Team (1996) Home versus hospital deliveries: follow up study of matched pairs for procedures and outcome. *BMJ*, 313, 1313–18.

BirthChoiceUK (2011) http://www.birthchoiceuk.com/ (accessed 16 March 2011).

Brown, A., Hall, H. and Mori, T. (2010) Presentation AM7: The Community Skills Day. 5th LSA National Conference for Supervisors of Midwives, Bradford Hospitals NHS Foundation Trust.

Chamberlain, G., Wraight, A., Crowley, P. (eds.) (1997) *Home Births* – The Report of the 1994 Confidential Enquiry by the National Birthday Trust (available in summary form at http://www.homebirth.org.uk/homebirth2.htm).

Centre for Maternal and Child Enquiries (CMACE) (2009) *The London Project: A Confidential Enquiry into a Series of Term Babies Born in an Unexpectedly Poor Condition.* The report commissioned by King's College Hospital (King's), is available on request from King's by email on: mediateam@kch.nhs.uk or by phone (0203 299 3257).

Centre for Maternal and Child enquiries (CMACE) (2011) *Saving Mother's Lives: Reviewing Maternal Deaths to Make Motherhood Safer: 2006–2008.* The Eighth Report on Confidential Enquiries into Maternal Deaths in the United Kingdom. *BJOG*, 118 (Suppl. 1), 1–203.

Department of Health (2007) *Maternity Matters: Choice, Access and Continuity of Care in a Safe Service.* London: Department of Health.

Gyte, G. and Dodwell, M. (2007) Safety of planned home birth: an NCT review of evidence. *New Digest*, 40, 20–9.

Janssen, P.A., Lee, S.K., Ryan, E.M., Etches, D.J., Farquarhson, D.F., Peacock, D. and Klein, M.C. (2002) Outcomes of planned home births versus planned hospital births after regulation of midwifery in British Columbia. *Canadian Medical Association Journal*, 166, 315–23.

de Jonge, A., van der Goes, B., Ravelli, A., Amelink-Verburg, M., Mol, B., Nijhuis, J., Bennebroek Gravenhorst, J. and Buitendijk, S. (2009) Perinatal mortality and morbidity in a nationwide cohort of 529 688 low-risk planned home and hospital births. *BJOG* (DOI: 10.1111/j.1471–0528.2009.02175.x).

Lewis, G. (ed.) (2007) The Confidential Enquiry into Maternal and Child Health (CEMACH). *Saving Mothers' Lives: Reviewing Maternal Deaths to Make Motherhood Safer – 2003–2005*. The Seventh Report on Confidential Enquiries into Maternal Deaths in the United Kingdom. London: CEMACH.

Local Supervising Authority (LSA) Midwifery Officers Forum (UK)/NMC (2009) *Modern Supervision in Action: A Practical Guide for Midwives*. London: NMC/LSAMO Forum (UK).

Local Supervising Authority (LSA) Midwifery Officers' Forum, UK (2010) www.midwife.org.uk (accessed 11 August 2010).

Madden, E. and McMechan, M. (2010) Presentation AM3: Supervision? Where's my lipstick? 5th LSA National Conference for Supervisors of Midwives (www.jmdevents.co.uk), South Eastern Health & Social Care Trust, Northern Ireland.

Midwifery 2020 (2010) *Delivering Expectations* (www.midwifery2020.org; accessed 17 March 2011).

Mori, R., Dougherty, M. and Whittle, M. (2008) An estimation of intrapartum-related perinatal mortality rates for booked home births in England and Wales between 1994 and 2003. *BJOG*, 115, 554–9.

NHS Litigation Authority (2010) Clinical Negligence Scheme for Trusts (CNST). *Maternity Clinical Risk Management Standards* Version 1 (http://www.nhsla.com/RiskManagement/; accessed 19 March 2011).

NHS Quality Improvement Scotland (2004) *Best Practice Statement on Maternal History Taking* (http://qualityimprovementscotland.com). Edinburgh: NHS Quality Improvement Scotland.

National Institute for Health and Clinical Excellence (2006) *Routine Postnatal Care of Women and Their Babies*. Clinical Guideline 37. London. National Collaborating Centre for Women's and Children's Health.

National Institute for Health and Clinical Excellence (2007) *Intrapartum Care*. Clinical Guideline 55. London: National Collaborating Centre for Women's and Children's Health.

National Institute for Health and Clinical Excellence (2008a) *Antenatal Care: Routine Care for the Healthy Pregnant Woman*. Clinical Guideline 62. London. National Collaborating Centre for Women's and Children's Health

National Institute for Health and Clinical Excellence (2008b) *Induction of Labour*. Clinical Guideline 70. London: National Collaborating Centre for Women's and Children's Health.

National Institute for Health and Clinical Excellence (2008c) *Routine Antenatal Anti-D Prophylaxis for Women who are Rhesus D Negative*. Technology Appraisal Guidance (TAG) 156. London: National Collaborating Centre for Women's and Children's Health.

Northern Health and Social Care Trust (2009) *Best Maternity Care Best Practice – a Strategy for the Maternity Service 2009–2014*. Northern Health and Social Care Trust (NI).

National Perinatal Epidemiology Unit (2010) https://npeu.ox.ac.uk/birthplace (accessed 17 March 2011).

Nursing and Midwifery Council (2004) *Midwives' Rules and Standards*. M/05/05 January 2005. London: Nursing and Midwifery Council.

Nursing and Midwifery Council (2006) Circular 8/2006. *Midwives and Homebirth*. London. Nursing and Midwifery Council.

Nursing and Midwifery Council (2007) *Standards for Medicines Management*. London: Nursing and Midwifery Council.

Nursing and Midwifery Council (2008) *The Code: Standards of Conduct, Performance and Ethics for Nurses and Midwives*. London: Nursing and Midwifery Council.

Nursing and Midwifery Council (2009a) *Record Keeping: Guidance for Nurses and Midwives*. London: Nursing and Midwifery Council.

Nursing and Midwifery Council (2009b) *Standards for Pre-registration Midwifery Education*. London: Nursing and Midwifery Council.

Nursing and Midwifery Council (2010a) *Advice and Information for Employers of Nurses and Midwives*. London: Nursing and Midwifery Council.

Nursing and Midwifery Council (2010b) *Support for Parents: How Supervision and Supervisors of Midwives Can Help You*. London: Nursing and Midwifery Council.

Nursing and Midwifery Council (2011) *Changes to Midwives' Exemptions*. Circular 07/2011. London: Nursing and Midwifery Council.

Olsen, O. and Jewell, D. (1998) Home versus hospital birth. *Cochrane Database of Systematic Reviews*, Issue 3, article no. CD000352 (DOI 10.1002/14651858.CD000352).

Royal College of Midwives (2002) *Home Birth Handbook, Vol. 1: Promoting Home Birth*. London: Royal College of Midwives.

Royal College of Midwives (2003) *Home Birth Handbook, Vol. 2: Practising Home Birth*. London: Royal College of Midwives.

Royal College of Obstetrics and Gynaecology (RCOG) (2010) *RCOG Statement on the King's Fund Discussion Paper on the Role of GPs in Maternity Care*. London. Royal College of Obstetrics and Gynaecology.

Royal College of Obstetrics and Gynaecology (RCOG), Royal College of Midwives, Royal College of Anaesthetists, and Royal College of Paediatrics and Child Health (2007) *Safer Childbirth: Minimum Standards for the Organisation and Delivery of Care in Labour*. London: Royal College of Obstetrics and Gynaecology.

Royal College of Obstetrics and Gynaecology/Royal College of Midwives (RCOG/RCM) (2007) Joint Statement Number 2. *Home Births*. London: RCOG/RCM.

Scottish Government (2011) *A Refreshed Framework for Maternity Care in Scotland: The Maternity Service Action Group*. Edinburgh: Scottish Government.

Walsh, D., El-Nemer, A. and Downe, S. (2004) Risk, safety and the study of physiological birth. In Downe, S. (ed.) *Normal Childbirth: The Evidence and the Debate*. Edinburgh: Churchill Livingstone.

Wax, J.R., Lucas, F.L., Lamont, M., Pinette, M.G., Cartin, A. and Blackstone, J. (2010) Maternal and newborn outcomes in planned home birth vs planned hospital births: a metaanalysis. *American Journal of Obstetrics and Gynecology*, 203(3), e8.

Woodcock, H.C., Read, A.W., Moore, D.J, Stanley, F.J. and Bower, C. (1990) Planned home-births in Western Australia 1981–1987: a descriptive study. *Medical Journal of Australia*, 153, 672–8.

Woodcock, H.C., Read, A.W., Bower, C., Stanley, F.J. and Moore, D.J. (1994) A matched cohort study of planned home and hospital births in Western Australia 1981–1987. *Midwifery*, 10, 125–35.

Appendix 3.1: When should I call the midwife?

Call the midwife any time day or night using the contact numbers if:

- you have any fresh red vaginal bleeding or clots;
- you are worried about reduced baby movements or anything else;
- your waters break and the fluid is clear, green, brown or has an offensive odour;
- you are having strong regular, painful contractions (remember that if you have had a baby before, your contractions may become stronger and closer together more quickly).

In addition:

- If you are planning to labour in water, call the midwife and await her arrival before you enter the pool.
- Your midwife may wish you to contact her when you think you are going into labour to allow her time to plan or get help with other work. You should discuss this with your midwife in advance.

Midwives' on-call contact details

Mobile
Landline
Base for midwife/team
Other (delivery suite/
    switchboard)

Appendix 3.2: Emergency callout

If an emergency happens, telephone 999 (or mobile 112) and say:

The midwife is requesting an emergency blue light ambulance with paramedic support for an obstetric emergency at a homebirth.

NAME:
(Of person(s) being transferred)

ADDRESS: Tel:
(With directions
and postcode)

SBAR

Situation: date, time, reason for transfer	Background: risk, diagnosis, treatment, relevant history, current condition
Assessment: airway, temperature, P, blood pressure, respiration, medication, fetal heart rate, progress, birth?, estimated blood loss?	Recommendation – *plan of care*

Name of midwife:
Date and time:
Signature:

Appendix 3.3: Notification of request for homebirth

To:_____ Community midwifery manager/team leader

I have received a request for a homebirth from:

Miss/Mrs/Ms *(delete)*	Date of birth:
Name:	Maternity no.:
	Hospital for transfer (if required):
	Interpreter required: yes/no
	Language:
Address:	GP:
	Health centre address:
Postcode:	
Tel no.:	Named midwife:
Mobile:	Base:
E-mail:	Tel no.:
Estimated date of delivery:	E-mail:
Gestation:	
Parity:	

Risk factors identified and discussed: YES ☐   NO ☐

Please list: _____

_____

_____

_____

Action plan: _____

_____

_____

_____

Signed: .... *(Midwife)*

Date: ....

Return completed form to community midwifery manager/team leader.
Insert a copy in woman's notes

Appendix 3.4: Notification of completed homebirth

To:_____ Community midwifery manager/team leader

I have attended a homebirth with:

Miss/Mrs/Ms *(delete)*	Date of birth:
Name:	Maternity no.:
	Hospital for transfer (if required):
	Interpreter required: yes/no
	Language:
Address:	GP:
	Health centre address:
Postcode:	
Tel no.:	Named midwife:
Mobile:	Base:
E-mail:	Tel no.:
Estimated date of delivery:	E-mail:
Gestation:	
Parity:	

Birth details	*Those present at birth*
Date of birth:	Midwife–birth
Time of birth:	
Male ☐ Female ☐	Midwife–baby
Gestational age: weeks+ days	
Apgar score	Birth partner:
at 1 minute	
at 5 minutes	
Computer data completed	Baby NHS or Health and Care No.:

Transferred to hospital care: YES ☐   NO ☐   Date:

Ambulance ☐   999 blue light ambulance ☐   Private transport ☐

Time ambulance called:

Time ambulance left house:

Time of arrival at hospital:

Reason for transfer:

Care handed over to:

Comments:

Signed: .... (*Midwife*)

Date: ....

Return completed form to community midwifery manager/team leader.
Insert a copy in the woman's notes.

Appendix 3.5: Birth plan for homebirth

Insert the birth plan at the front of the maternity hand held record

Name:	Maternity services no.:
Address:	Date of birth:
Postcode:	Estimated date of delivery:
	Number of children:
Tel no.:	GP:

Housekeeping arrangements

Room in the home where the birth is likely to take place: _____

Room heater ❐   Good source of lighting ❐   Emergency access to home ❐

If there are house pets, arrangements to be made for their care

Sanitary facilities including toilet and hot water facilities

Birth partners

Who is going to be present during labour? _____

_____

_____

Names and ages of other children: _____

_____

_____

Who is taking care of your child/children during labour? _____

_____

_____

Who will help and support you immediately following birth?_____

_____

_____

First stage of labour

Moving around, eating a light diet and drinking normally during labour are encouraged.

Managing during labour:

Do you plan to use (tick all that apply):
Mobility ☐   Aromatherapy oils ☐
Alternative positions ☐   TENS ☐
Water ☐   Entonox ☐
Music ☐
Other: _____

Monitoring the baby's heartbeat:

May the midwife use a Sonicaid?   YES ☐   NO ☐
A Pinard stethoscope?   YES ☐   NO ☐

Second stage of labour

What position do you want to be in to give birth to your baby?

_____

_____

Do you want your baby lifted on to your tummy?   YES ☐   NO ☐

_____

_____

Who do you wish to cut the cord?   YES ☐   NO ☐
Comments: _____

_____

Third stage of labour – delivery of placenta and membranes (ask your midwife for details)

Do you plan to have 'physiological' management of third stage? *(no medicines)*
YES ☐   NO ☐

Do you plan to have 'active' management? *(includes injection)*
YES ☐   NO ☐
Do you give your permission for the midwife to use an oxytocic medicine in an emergency?   YES ☐   NO ☐

After the birth

Are you happy to have:
Early skin-to-skin contact   YES ☐   NO ☐
Early breast-feeding   YES ☐   NO ☐

The midwife will examine your baby from head to toe.
When can the midwife weigh the baby? _____
_____

Students

Do you give your permission for a student to be present during pregnancy, childbirth and afterwards?   YES ☐   NO ☐

Concerns and transfer

If the midwife has any clinical concerns about you or your baby do you consent to being transferred to an appropriate hospital for further care?
YES ☐   NO ☐
_____
_____

Will your birth partner have access to transport to/from hospital if necessary?
YES ☐   NO ☐

Any other comments or requests?
_____
_____
_____
_____

Reasons for giving my newborn baby vitamin K have been clearly explained to me and I have received a copy of the vitamin K leaflet
YES ☐   NO ☐

I give consent for my baby to have vitamin K at birth in accordance with the current local policy (please select and delete below)
by injection ☐
or orally × 3 doses ☐
or I do not give consent for my baby to have vitamin K ☐

Signed: _____ (woman) Date: _____

Signed: _____ (midwife) Date: _____

Woman's checklist for homebirth

SOME SUGGESTIONS TO HELP YOU PREPARE FOR THE BIRTH OF YOUR BABY

Midwife on-call rota

Maternity records

Medicines as discussed with the midwife

Paracetamol

Vitamin K (one or three ampoules)

Prescription needed?

Secure locked box/cupboard for the safe storage of medicines (if required)

Midwife contact details

Medical gases

Oxygen for mother (tubing, masks)

Oxygen for baby (tubing, masks)

Entonox cylinders

Other ....

Local guidelines for safe storage of equipment, medical gases and medicines (if required)

Home: essential requirements

Telephone access

Room heater

Good light source and torch

Protective covers for bed and floor

Disposable pads or 'old' clean towels or sheets

Extra pillows with plastic covers

Padded surface at table height

Pint/litre jug with markings

Sponge or flannel

Digital thermometer

Optional

TENS

Fan

Aromatherapy or other complementary therapy – please consult a qualified therapist

Hot water bottle and cover or wheat pack covered

Mother

Sanitary maternity towels

Breastfeeding bras

Old loose nightie/shirt

Disposable/old pants

Warm socks

Fluids, e.g. fruit/isotonic drinks

Bendy straws

Glucose sweets

Snacks/easily digested food

Lip moisturiser

Hair bobble

Background music

Camera/film

Packed bag for emergencies

Baby

Vest

Cardigans

Babygros

Socks

Hat

Mittens

Cot/basket

Sheets and blankets

Newborn nappies

Baby bath

For midwife

Hot water

Soap

Hand towels

Appendix 3.6: Suggested equipment for midwives' homebirth kit

Carried by midwifery staff
Mobile phone or bleeper
Baby scales
Sphygmomanometer, stethoscope
Sonicaid (with spare gel and battery)
Pinard stethoscope
Body temperature thermometer
Watch with second hand
Spare black pens
Antiseptic hand wipes or gel

Medicines – midwives' exemptions
Diclofenac suppository
Vitamin K, 2 mg (0.2 ml) × three ampoules
Syntometrine 1 ml × two ampoules
Ergometrine 500 µg × two ampoules
Lidocaine 1% (20 ml) × two ampoules

Hospital pharmacy
Aquagel sachets

GP prescriptions
Ranitidine 150 mg × three tablets

Medical gases from hospital or community pharmacy
For medical gases check if integrated head is attached
Oxygen – two small cylinders, size CD (integral heads), tubing
Entonox – four small cylinders, size CD (integral heads), tubing – or two large cylinders: size F, and one detachable head, tubing and two trolleys
Cylinder wrenches if detached heads
Entonox filter, mouthpiece and mask
Trolleys for medical gases

Homebirth bag
Gloves (various sizes, sterile/ non-sterile, non-latex)
Tape measure (disposable)
Multistix
Microbiology swabs (×4)
Disposable scissors
Surface wipes – alco-wipes and soap and water wipes
Spare cord clamps (×3)
Water thermometer
Torch and battery

Venepuncture equipment
Spot plasters and cotton wool balls
Blood bottles
Vacutainer/syringes
Needles
Sharps box
Rhesus negative pack
Forms for cord bloods
Blood bottles for rhesus negative

Additional disposable equipment
Placenta disposal box with lid
Yellow bags
Black bags
Black identifier tags for bags
Aprons
Emesis bowls (×3)
Plastic covers (×2)
Spare sanitary pads
Absorbable pads
Disposable bedpan

Neonatal resuscitation bag
Portable suction machine
Ambubag, paediatric
Oxygen tubing
Facemasks (two paediatric sizes)
Infant airways: sizes 00 and 000
Suction catheters (mini-Yanker)
Orange needles (×4)
Syringes (1 and 2 ml)

Intrapartum equipment
Delivery pack and instrument tray
Sterile cotton wool balls, gauze squares
Suturing tray and material (×2)
Tampons (×3)
Sterile drape (×2)
Disposable speculum
Goggles
Amnistix (×4)
Catheterisation pack (×3)
In–out catheter (×3)
Mid-stream urine bottle

Adult resuscitation bag
Adult airways sizes 2, 3 and 4
Yanker suction
Oxygen tubing
Adult oxygen mask
Adult Ambubag
Suction tubing

Documents
Homebirth operational
　guidelines
Maternity hand held record
On-call rota with contact
　telephone numbers
PCHR (Red Book) (boy/girl)
Notification of birth form
Notification of completion of
　birth (if used locally)
Newborn hearing test
　information leaflet
Vitamin K information leaflet
Neonatal bloodspot
　information leaflet
BCG questionnaire and
　information
Microbiology forms

Chapter 4   **Supporting homebirth**

Mary Steen and Kath Jones

Introduction

This chapter will focus on supporting homebirth and will commence by examining antenatal preparation and the importance of 'being with woman'. Promoting childbirth without fear is an important aspect of care. How this can positively influence women to believe in their ability to give birth normally, have the confidence to do so and consider having the birth in their own home will be discussed. The debate whether there is a difference between poor and better health and well-being outcomes associated with place of birth is included. Midwives play a vital role in promoting and influencing normal birth practices; therefore this chapter will explore and discuss how midwives support women to make informed decisions about their birth place choices.

Preparing partners and a homebirth plan of care which covers both the woman's and midwife's perspective are important aspects to consider; these are necessary to promote good communication between the woman, her family, the midwife and the maternity services. It is essential for midwives to know and be familiar with the local procedures and systems in place for registering a request for homebirth, the equipment and documentation required. It is important that the expectant mother and partner or other attending person knows how to call a midwife when in labour or in an emergency if the need arises. These aspects are, therefore, included to enable midwives to provide high standards of care when supporting women requesting homebirths.

> Home birth requires practitioners who are able to watch, wait and be patient.
>
> (Davies, 2004, p. 154)

Antenatal preparation

During the antenatal period, it is important that women receive information and guidance about normal birth practices and their birth environment choices. The majority of women are deemed 'low risk' and therefore homebirth is an option that should be offered. Yet in the UK homebirth rates remain low, approximately 2.69 per cent (BirthChoice UK, 2009a).

Working in partnership with the woman and involving her partner, a midwife can actively reduce a woman's 'fear of childbirth'. Reducing fear and promoting normal birth practices will empower women to consider homebirth as an option. Increasing awareness of the choice of homebirth and good preparation during pregnancy will help some women to have a homebirth.

Good preparation for homebirth will:

- increase women's knowledge of the risks and benefits of opting for a homebirth;
- help expectant fathers to support their partner during the homebirth;
- reduce the likelihood of interventions during labour and childbirth;
- reduce the analgesic types of pain relief;
- increase the number of women being active during childbirth;
- increase the number of fathers adopting an active/supportive role during childbirth;
- increase the number of women and their partners having a positive birth experience.

A midwife can encourage and enable a woman, firstly, to believe in her ability to give birth normally; secondly, to gain the courage and confidence to do so; and, thirdly, to view homebirth as a viable option. Midwives, however, may need to reflect on their clinical practice and skills and ask themselves if they are truly 'being with woman' (Figure 4.1).

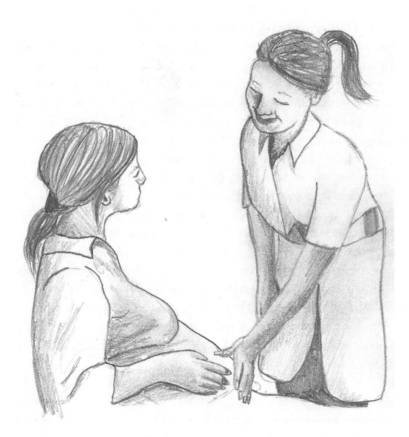

FIGURE 4.1 Pregnant woman and midwife (touching the pregnant womb).

Being with woman

No one is going to dispute that for many women giving birth is intensely physical and emotional and that during labour their care is based on individual needs (Steen and Calvert, 2007). However, how we provide care and support to women needs to be reflected upon. Has the dominant medical model of care influenced midwives' views of women's ability to give birth normally and women's options for a homebirth?

Davis-Floyd (2001) suggests that the aim to give holistic care may be too great a challenge in institutions that are technologically orientated, owing to the authoritative knowledge suppressing other ways of knowing. Walsh and Steen (2007) highlight the need to review the role of the midwife and practice setting. They identify four key areas that need to be taken into consideration to enable midwives to promote normal birth and homebirth as a choice: autonomy, normality, holism and woman-centredness.

Physical and emotional support during labour has been shown to be beneficial, and there is evidence that one-to-one support in labour does have a beneficial effect on normal birth outcomes (Sandall, 2004). A Cochrane systematic review has provided evidence that emotional support, information and advice can promote normal birth (Hodnett *et al.*, 2011). Another Cochrane systematic review compared care in a 'home-like birth environment' with care in a 'conventional labour ward' and found evidence that birth in 'home-like setting' had health benefits and significantly increase the likelihood of no intrapartum analgesia/anaesthesia being required (Hodnett *et al.*, 2010).

If a 'home-like setting' has health benefits, then surely the real thing has? 'There is no place like home' (Gwillim, 2009, p. 83). At home a woman is familiar with her surroundings, and this can make her feel less anxious and fearful; she is less likely to be restricted and will remain active during labour. Basically, she is in control of her own environment in which to give birth (Kitzinger, 2002). She will have one-to-one support from a midwife and, more than likely, her partner will take an active role. Hunter (2005) found that midwives working in community settings were better able to work in a 'with woman' model of care that fitted their philosophy of midwifery. Interestingly, there is evidence that in remote Inuit villages in Canada, where healthy women labour in their own communities supported by midwives, perinatal outcomes are similar to, and sometimes better than, Canadian outcomes as a whole (van Wagner, 2007).

Yet in developed countries, where there is good access to medical care and skilled health professionals who attend homebirths, there appears to be a focus on the risks that can happen during labour and childbirth, and the benefits do not seem to be given equal weighting. Home versus hospital birth environment is an on-going debate, and evidence to confirm or refute which is the safest place remains inconclusive (National Perinatal Epidemiology Unit, 2010).

The debate

Let us not forget that home is the natural place to give birth and at the end of pregnancy women innately 'nest' and prepare for the forthcoming birth of their infant. However, in the twentieth century the shift from home to hospital and the increasing medicalisation of childbirth has influenced how birth is viewed and experienced (see Chapter 1). Stephens (2005) found that many women and their partners believe hospital is the safest place to give birth and homebirth is unsafe. Therefore, the majority of women will give birth in a hospital setting (consultant-led unit), but women do have other choices.

In the UK, the Department of Health (2007) recommends that all women are advised about their birth choices and can choose their home, a consultant-led unit or birth centre. A woman's birth place choices should be discussed with her first at the antenatal booking appointment and then again later on in pregnancy, and it should be made clear that it is a choice and she can change her mind at any time. Women who are identified as high risk will be advised to deliver their baby in a consultant-led unit. Most women with an identified problem that could put her baby or herself at increased risk will choose this option. However, if a woman does not, a midwife has a 'statutory duty' to provide care and support women who choose to have a homebirth regardless of whether she is deemed low or high risk (Nursing and Midwifery Council, 2004).

In Scotland, the *Framework for Maternity Services in Scotland* (Scottish Executive Health Department, 2001) and the *Report of the Expert Group on Acute Maternity Services* (Scottish Executive Health Department, 2002) endorsed the promotion of pregnancy and childbirth as normal life events. They recommended community-focused, midwife-led care for healthy women experiencing uncomplicated pregnancies, and multidisciplinary maternity team care for women with more complexity. The Keeping Childbirth Natural and Dynamic (KCND) programme has been developed to promote multiprofessional partnership working and implement a traffic light system approach for women and babies based on need (NHS Quality Improvement Scotland, 2009).

In April 2004, the 'All Wales Clinical Pathway for Normal Labour' was introduced and implemented throughout Wales. This clinical pathway was developed to reduce unnecessary medical intervention and promote normal labour and birth; it has helped to promote and increase homebirth as a choice for women in Wales (NHS Wales, 2006; see also Appendix 4.1).

Position statements and guidelines can be very helpful but can also have their limitations and obstetric biases. The Royal College of Midwives (RCM) and the Royal College of Obstetricians and Gynaecologists (RCOG)

> support homebirth for women with uncomplicated pregnancies. There is no reason why homebirth should not be offered to women at low risk of complications, and it may confer considerable benefits for them and their families. There is ample evidence showing that labouring at home increases a woman's likelihood of a birth that is both satisfying and safe, with implications for her health and that of her baby.
>
> (RCOG/RCM, 2007)

In contrast, the Royal Australian and New Zealand College of Obstetricians and Gynaecologists (RANZCOG) appears to be specifically risk focused and do not take into consideration the benefits of birthing at home (RANZCOG, 2009). The College will not endorse a woman's choice to have a homebirth, owing to concerns raised about large geographical distances to the nearest consultant-led units. However, the provision of maternity services in local communities is complex; economic reasons and workforce shortages have contributed to a lack of provision to provide a homebirth service.

In the UK, geographical distances are not generally a cause for concern, but an increasing birth rate, more complex cases and financial and staffing problems have had an effect on maternity service provision, and some units have had to activate an 'escalation' policy and close. This has had a knock-on effect on midwives being able to attend homebirths. To counteract this, some maternity services have introduced homebirth teams. O'Connell and colleagues (2011) have recently reported positive feedback from women and also a significant increase in the number of homebirths attended since a home-birth team was established by Northampton General Hospital NHS Trust. This homebirth team won the RCM 2011 midwifery award for implementing government policy. In some areas, independent midwives are successfully gaining contracts to provide midwifery care and support homebirth provision (Independent Midwives UK, 2011).

In Australia, the closure of rural maternity units has left many Australian women with little choice but to plan their birth within a consultant-led unit. Transportation time is a significant factor in safety, yet there appears to be no recognition of the risks of road travel for a labouring woman. A recent qualitative study of the experiences of women and some of their partners in New South Wales, Australia, found that the risk of dangerous road travel, and the deprivations experienced when women labour en route, are ignored in obstetric risk discourse (Dietsch *et al.*, 2010). Many women questioned why they needed to risk unsafe road travel when their preference was to labour and birth in their local communities with a midwife. Nevertheless, the risk-averse obstetric culture does not appear to have improved perinatal birth outcomes for women in Australia (Australian Institute of Health and Welfare, 2003; Hancock, 2007).

In the USA, the American Medical Association (2008) and the American College of Obstetricians and Gynaecologists (2008) also oppose homebirth on the basis that a seemingly uncomplicated birth can still potentially become a medical emergency without warning. There appears to be an assumption that a hospital where surgeons and anaesthetists are available is the safest place to give birth. Yet, as emphasised earlier in this book, 'absolute safety for women in birth cannot be assured at home, in a midwifery-led unit or in hospital and all places may have risks attached' (see Chapter 2, 'Safety of homebirth'). A recently updated Cochrane review continues to conclude what the authors reported in their first issue in the late 1990s: there is no strong evidence to favour either home or hospital birth for low-risk pregnant women (Olsen and Jewell, 1998).

A national cohort study undertaken in the Netherlands concluded that homebirth does not increase the risks of perinatal mortality and severe peri-natal morbidity among low-risk women, provided the maternity care system facilitates this choice through the availability of well-trained midwives and through a good transportation and referral system (de Jonge *et al.*, 2009). However, this study has been criticised because the findings may not be rep-resentative of other populations and, as the data collected relied upon the accuracy of recording all outcomes within national databases, there may be some error in data entry or missed information (NHS Knowledge, 2009).

Recently, Wax and colleagues (2010) carried out a meta-analysis in the USA and reported that planned homebirths, when compared with planned hospi-tal births, were associated with fewer maternal interventions, less maternal morbidity and less analgesic use. This meta-analysis also found a significant increase in neonatal mortality rates with planned homebirths and concluded that less medical intervention and morbidity associated with planned home-births must be weighed against the significant increase in neonatal mortality rates. However, this review of the evidence and analysis has been heavily criticised and serious methodological limitations have been highlighted (Gyte *et al.*, 2010). A lack of information about the included studies, the quality assessment criteria and the data contributed by these studies was highlighted.

Numerous letters were sent to the editors of the *American Journal of Obstetrics and Gynecology* regarding this article (Anon., 2011). In response to the concerns that were expressed in the letters, an independent review was undertaken. Additional information was requested, which included the individual summary graphs for each outcome that was presented. The independent reviewers focused on the 'numbers' that were included for each outcome in the meta-analysis. The results were found to be slightly different from the result published. However, there was no difference reported in the direction of the point estimate of the pooled odds ratio or in the overall 'statistical significance' of the results. It was recommended that the journal publish online full summary graphs for each outcome that was assessed in the study, to give readers an opportunity to assess the study findings in greater detail, and no retraction of the article was deemed necessary.

The letters raised a number of issues regarding the methodological limitations of the meta-analysis and why some studies were excluded. The reviewers believed that some of the issues commented upon were subjective and should therefore be debated openly.

The evidence to confirm or refute whether place of birth is associated with health outcomes remains inconclusive. For this reason, the 'Birth Place in England Research Programme' has been commissioned by the National Institute for Health Research (NIHR) and the Department of Health (National Perinatal Epidemiology Unit, 2010). This research programme will compare outcomes of births planned at home, in different types of midwifery units and in consultant-led units.

However, the heart of the problem is that the NHS is structured to deal only with 'patients' and 'visitors', not with a natural family event such as a birth (Fisher, 2009). Therefore, it is not too surprising that many women's birth experience remains highly medicalised in the western world. Labour is managed and time constraints are enforced. Birth often takes place in an unfamiliar, often intimidating, hospital environment with machinery, limited space to move around and lack of one-to-one care (Steen and Walsh, 2007). Boucher and colleagues (2009) have reported that many expectant mothers choose homebirth as they want to deliver in their own familiar surroundings. Others choose homebirth because they dislike a hospital environment. Yet Sheila Kitzinger has highlighted that many more women want homebirths than actually are able to for lack of support: 'Women who make the decision to give birth at home must usually overcome many obstacles put in place by the medical system' (Kitzinger, 2000, p. 11).

There is evidence emerging that birth in the twenty-first century for many women is having detrimental effects on their health and well-being (Simpkin, 1991; Emerson, 1998; Murphy et al., 2003). This leads to the question concerning how risk relating to birth is assessed and evaluated. Basically, the risks associated with birth are an estimation of the probability of something happening. This is based on a clinical assessment of a woman's past and present health and well-being status and the identification of predisposing factors that will indicate her estimated risk of an event occurring. The woman is categorised as being at 'high' or 'low' risk. This risk management approach is not entirely effective, and risk scoring systems should be regarded with caution (Ekin *et al.*, 2000). Some women considered to be 'low' risk may still have unexpected complications, and some women considered to be 'high' risk may turn out to have an uneventful pregnancy and birth. As with all life events there will always be an element of uncertainty and unpredictability.

However, it is important to consider how the woman views these risks. For example, case study 6 in Chapter 8, 'Homebirth – waterbirth', describes and discusses how a woman with multiple sclerosis is categorised as 'high' risk but she does not consider herself to be high risk:

> I'm in remission and feel fit and well. Yes, I struggle with walking and sometimes have to use a stick but I cannot see any reason why I cannot have a waterbirth at home as I use hydrotherapy frequently to ease my joint pains . . . after all the appointments and treatments I have received over the last few years I have a fear of going anywhere near a hospital.

Does the risk of her fear of hospitals and how this may affect her birth experience outweigh the identified risk of her having a medical disorder? This woman made the decision that it does and a homebirth would minimise this risk. Her views were considered and she was supported to have a homebirth, but how many women are not? Physical, emotional/psychological, social and environmental risk factors need to be considered when undertaking a risk assessment. This will help to reduce the risk of the detrimental effects associated with birth upon women's health and well-being that have been recently reported.

Legal regulations in some western countries can also play a part in inhibiting a woman's choice to have a homebirth. Although homebirths are legal, in many western countries insurance either is too expensive or does not cover midwives to attend. In the UK, there is no professional indemnity insurance available for independent midwives, and therefore independent midwives are personally liable in the event of a negligence claim. The Nursing and Midwifery Council requires independent midwives to inform all women that they do not have professional indemnity insurance and the implications of this. Midwives employed by the NHS are covered through their trusts and have the Clinical Negligence Scheme for Trusts (CNST), which is governed by the NHS Litigation Authority (NHSLA).

Controversy is presently on-going in Hungary. The European Court of Human rights has criticised the 'permanent threat' to health professionals in Hungary who attend homebirths. In a recent case brought to the court by a Hungarian woman (Ternovszky *v.* Hungary) the court upheld the woman's right to choose where to give birth, and decreed that Article 8 of the European Convention (right to private and family life) had been violated (European Court of Human Rights, 2010) (see Appendix 4.2). Recently, a bill was passed in the Republic of Hungary to legalise homebirth as of 1 May 2011, but midwives are being refused certification to attend, and those who do attend homebirths are under severe scrutiny. Agnes Gereb, an obstetrician and midwife who has been supporting women to have homebirths for the last 20 years, was arrested in October 2010 on criminal charges allegedly associated with homebirths (Hill, 2010). The RCM supports the release of Agnes Gereb and for the introduction of legislation in Hungary which would allow midwives to perform out-of-hospital births. The RCM calls on the Hungarian authorities to urgently address these issues (see Appendix 4.3). On 24 March 2011, the Budapest Court of Justice found Agnes guilty of endangering life in the pursuit of her professional duties; another midwife was fined and three others were acquitted. Agnes has been sentenced to two years' imprisonment and debarred from practising as a midwife for five years. International experts on homebirth disagree with this judgment and are lobbying for her release. She is presently appealing this decision.

Some women, for these reasons, are choosing to 'birth alone', which has become known as 'freebirthing'. Freebirthing is not illegal in the UK, but it is illegal for a partner, family member or friend to intentionally plan to replace a skilled professional at the birth. Some reasons given by women who are choosing to 'birth alone' are that the NHS maternity services are failing to meet their birth needs and they often feel coerced into a birth that is far removed from what they want and desire (Cooper and Clarke, 2008).

Recently, the media reported the case of a woman who chose to freebirth in Bulgaria and whose baby unfortunately died. This was her second pregnancy and she had decided not to go into hospital in an attempt to avoid invasive medical procedures and to have a normal birth (Sofia News Agency, 2011).

Nolan (2011, p. 113) suggests that 'free birthing is a form of social protest' and it 'provides an opportunity for the maternity service to reflect on whether it is meeting women's needs as comprehensively as it can'.

The Royal College of Midwives in the UK recognises these problems and has recently commissioned midwifery researchers to review and update the latest available evidence regarding midwifery-led models of care (Devane *et al.*, 2010). A comprehensive review that included a systematic review, meta-analysis, meta-synthesis and an economic analysis was undertaken, and the findings led the RCM to launch a new campaign to promote midwife-led care and its benefits. A published report of these findings can be downloaded from the RCM website. The Department of Health has published several reports to support the promotion of normal birth practices and give women choices of where to give birth (Department of Health, 2004, 2007, 2010). However, change does not happen overnight and the presence of a dominant medical model of childbirth throughout the western world will take time to change.

That said, homebirth should be promoted to all low-risk expectant mothers in countries where it is possible to establish a homebirth service backed up by a good hospital system (Olsen and Jewell, 1998). As Lord Hunt (2000) stated, 'if a woman wishes to have a homebirth she should receive the appropriate support from the health service. At the end of the day, it must be the woman's choice.'

Childbirth without fear

In most spontaneous labours, everything will occur as nature planned. Hormones associated with labour and birth are secreted to help labour progress steadily and safely. In 'normal' labour, the uterine muscles contract as they should, there is no cephalopelvic disproportion and women have the ability to manage their birth. However, fear in uncomplicated births can lead to an increase in the release of adrenaline, leading to excessive muscle tension, and this in turn can cause an increase in the severity of pain experienced by a woman to such an extent that it can become unbearable (Alehagen *et al.*, 2005). Fear can be acquired by suggestion or association and can manifest itself in dread and dismay, even terror, depending on the nature of the stimulus and a person's personality (Tucker, 2003).

For centuries childbirth has been accepted as a dangerous and painful experience. Civilisation, cultural beliefs and complicated births have influenced how birth is viewed. The bible teachings have instilled a generic fear of childbirth, and the 'Curse of Eve' has given women a reason to fear birth: 'Unto the woman he said, I will greatly multiply thy sorrow and thy conception; in sorrow thou shalt bring forth children' (Genesis 3:16).

And this was indeed the case for many women over the centuries, until the great advances of science and living conditions played their role in improving the health and well-being of women and thus reducing maternal and fetal mortality rates.

It is not too surprising that pain associated with labour and birth is feared by many women. Frye (2004, p. 258) states, 'western culture is probably about as afraid of pain as it is of death, both of which are issues that the pregnant and birthing woman must confront directly as she prepares to give birth and become a mother'. No doubt great advances in the care of expectant mothers and their babies have contributed to better maternal and fetal outcomes, but fear has impacted on how women view and experience childbirth.

Ina May Gaskin (2008, p. 149) gives some good advice: 'We need to always remember that mothers who are afraid tend to secrete the hormones that delay or inhibit birth'. Grantly Dick-Read (1959), in his famous book *Childbirth without Fear*, describes and discusses how he ploughed through mud and rain on his bicycle in the early hours to attend a woman living in poverty in the Whitechapel area of London. The home conditions were appalling, yet a sense of tranquillity and calm were clearly apparent. Dick-Read tried to persuade the woman to breathe in some chloroform as the baby's head crowned. She refused this firmly and there was no fuss or noise when the baby was born. This surprised Dick-Read as his experience of attending women in labour was that they needed pain relief.

> I have often wondered if a woman in Whitechapel whose name I have long since forgotten has ever realised the far-reaching influence of a casual remark she made to me, 'It didn't hurt. It wasn't meant to was it, doctor?'
> (Dick-Read, 2004, p. 23)

Many years afterwards, Dick-Read observed that some women have relatively painless childbirth experiences while others suffer intense pain. Many of these births resulted in a normal delivery even though the mother's experience could be described as horrible. Dick-Read recognised that it was the tranquil calm environment and state of mind of the labouring woman that influenced her birthing experience. Some women appeared to have faith in their ability to give birth and did so calmly and in control. 'So why, then, does it hurt?' asked Dick-Read, and he came up with the fear–tension–pain syndrome.

Fear of childbirth

When a woman fears childbirth she becomes anxious and fearful. Her body will tense up and become rigid during her labour. Her perception of pain will increase and she will experience excessive pain in her groin, round her lower back and down her legs. She will become tired and weary. This is a natural physical response to her anxiety and fear. Yet she will not be progressing in labour, her cervix not dilating and the labour pains ineffective. She will become increasingly frustrated and tearful and will ask for pain relief (Steen and Walsh, 2007).

Fear is a complex emotion that will bring resistant actions and reactions to the progress of labour. Fear will promote the natural protective mechanisms in a woman's body and muscle tension is created. The physical tensions that fear can cause will then interfere with the actions of the uterine muscle fibres, restrict the blood supply and hence have an impact on the effectiveness of labour contractions. Many women will not progress and will, therefore, become increasingly more anxious and afraid and be caught up in a vicious cycle of fear, tension and pain. Fear and anxiety increases emotional tension, and this will lead to the release of adrenaline, which will also increase the severity of pain perceived during labour.

In the twenty-first century this is a common phenomenon, and reducing this generic fear in women is a high priority for midwives to tackle, particularly in western countries, where increasingly the medical model of care has changed the culture of birth. This fear of childbirth has had an effect on women's confidence and ability to give birth normally, and this has influenced their birth environment choice.

The majority of women in the UK now give birth in a hospital environment, but a small percentage has the option of a birth centre and the choice of homebirth is available, but how well this choice is promoted and resources made available to ensure that it is a viable option remains questionable.

There is evidence that many women are anxious and even depressed during pregnancy and become fretful around the time of birth and actually fear birth itself (Brockington, 1998; Melender, 2002). A lack of understanding of the normal physiological process of birth, poor preparation for birth, lack of support and increasing use of technology has contributed to this fearful childbirth phenomenon (Steen and Walsh, 2007).

> When it comes to the culture of fear around birth, we are all in this together and we can only get out of it together.
>
> (Fisher, 2009)

Reducing fear is an extremely important goal during labour and birth. The physical and emotional needs of the woman have to be addressed. Continuity of care and being supported can reduce levels of fear and promote normal birth.

> Those who are not terrified are more likely to secrete in abundance the hormones that make labor and birth easier and less painful.
>
> (Gaskin, 2008, p. 149)

To counteract this fear of childbirth and reduce unnecessary medical intervention the RCM has set up a 'Campaign for Normal Birth' (Royal College of Midwives, 2005).

Normal birth

It is reasonable to assume that the promotion of normal birth and midwifery skills are strongly associated with the principles of a social model of care.

Promoting normal birth practices in the twenty-first century is a huge challenge and cultural change for maternity services.

Interestingly, Dick-Read (1959) stated:

> It is possible to say that labour has not yet become established and it is possible to say that labour is now well established but it is never possible to say that at a certain time in minutes even hours, labour actually commenced.

And according to RCOG/RCM (2007, p. 1), 'Birth for a woman is a rite of passage and a family life event, as well as being the start of a lifelong relationship with her baby'. These statements support the need to adopt a social model of care approach to support the normal physiological process of birth which can safely take place in the home environment.

Social model versus medical model

In recent years, Davis-Floyd (2001) and Walsh and Newburn (2002) have contrasted the values and beliefs underpinning the medical model of care with those from a social model (Table 4.1).

Although it would be wrong to stereotype individuals and maternity services as wholly one model or the other, it is helpful to articulate their primary orientation using these models (Steen and Walsh, 2007).

TABLE 4.1 Medical and social model of care compared

Medical	Social
Body as machine	Whole person
Reductionism – powers, passages, passenger	Integrate – physiology, psychosocial, spiritual
Control and subjugate	Respect and empower
Expertise/objective	Relational/subjective
Environment peripheral	Environment central
Anticipate pathology	Anticipate normality
Technology as master	Technology as servant
Homogenisation	Celebrate difference
Evidence	Intuition
Safety	Self-actualisation

International Confederation of Midwives (ICM)

ICM supports normal childbirth in countries as, for the majority of women, pregnancy and childbirth are physiological life events. Women should have access to midwifery-led care, one-to-one support and interdisciplinary working, including the choice of a homebirth and immersion in water. Midwifery associations must influence and work in collaboration with their ministries of health and other organisations. Note that the term 'childbirth' here encompasses pregnancy, birth and the postnatal period.

ICM supports the following definition of normal childbirth:

> Normal birth is where the woman commences, continues and completes labour with the infant being born spontaneously at term, with cephalic birth presentation, without any surgical, medical, or pharmaceutical intervention, but with the possibility of referral when needed.
> (International Confederation of Midwives, 2008, p. 1)

Normal birth practices

To promote normal birth, it is important that women receive information about normal birth practices for women often 'choose' to do what is expected of them and the most common image of the labouring woman is lying on the bed. Lying down continues to remain the most common position in labour. Midwives, therefore, need to be proactive in demonstrating and encouraging different positions in labour. Women should be encouraged and helped to move and adopt whatever positions they find most comfortable throughout labour (National Institute for Health and Clinical Excellence, 2007).

Campaign for Normal Birth

This Campaign for Normal Birth 'aims to inspire and support normal birth practice to maximise opportunities for women to experience normal birth and to reduce unnecessary medical intervention' (Royal College of Midwives, 2005). According to statistics quoted by BirthChoice UK (2009a), only 47 per cent of women in England, 38 per cent in Scotland and 39 per cent in Wales and Northern Ireland give birth without intervention. More recent statistics show that homebirth rates remain relatively low: England 2.69 per cent, Wales 3.83 per cent, Scotland 1.47 per cent, North Ireland 0.37 per cent. The RCM is very concerned that child-bearing women and maternity care professionals have become more dependent on technology in labour and birth.

The campaign is underpinned by the RCM's philosophy of pregnancy and birth as normal physiological processes, with a commitment to a positive reduction in unnecessary medicalisation, as outlined in Vision 2000 (Royal College of Midwives, 2000).

Vision 2000 was the forerunner for this campaign. The vision outlined 12 key points to enhance the adaptation of a social model of care, choice and continuity of care and to promote normal birth for all women:

- a service which listens to women;
- a focus on public health;
- a community orientation;
- integration across acute and community sectors;
- normality;
- midwifery-led care;
- maximised and targeted continuity of carer;
- dedicated one-to-one midwifery care in labour;
- family-centred care;
- clinical excellence;
- midwifery leadership;
- partnership.

A website has been developed to promote positive birth stories as a means to address the big issues to do with normal birth. At the heart of the campaign are useful tips, themes and stories to help midwives gain confidence in their ability to promote normal birth. See http://www.rcmnormalbirth.net/ for more information.

Balancing the art and science of midwifery is at the forefront of the RCM's campaign for normal birth. Midwives need to use a range of cognitive, psychomotor and emotive skills to fulfil their caring role. A midwife will need to have developed skills for 'sussing out labour', 'recognise her intuitive skills' and 'know how to work with pain' rather than just offering pain relief methods. These skills are important aspects of care that will promote normal birth (Steen and Walsh, 2007).

Midwives' skills

Skills for 'sussing out' labour

Midwives will use a combination of skills to 'suss out' labour. These include finely tuned observation of bodily and psychological processes, previous experience, gut instinct and research evidence. The ability to trust normal physiological processes and give individualised care to women is clearly defined in labour care. Habitually, health professionals have focused upon linear progress in labour, but recent research and a better understanding of birth hormones has revealed variations in labour patterns as physiological (Albers *et al.*, 1999; Buckley, 2005). This understanding of labour calls into question the necessity for repeated vaginal examination and opens up the possibility of reading these variations intuitively.

Intuition of the midwife

Intuition as a skill is probably a combination of accrued experience and unspoken knowledge that is hard to articulate. Bastick (1982) has reported that intuition involves a sudden immediacy of awareness that is often accompanied by emotions, a sense of certainty and predisposition to 'all is well' or 'something is amiss'.

Narrative research exploring birth stories undertaken by Ólafsdóttir (2010) describes how a midwife thinks this is an art: 'I often think about this as an art form, thinking as an artist painting who thinks, – no this is not right like this, it should be otherwise or something – you know.'

It is likely that the development of intuition requires appraising and reappraising in the light of experience and is often undermined by over-reliance on technology and prescriptive protocols.

Working with pain

One area where intuitive reading of a situation is clearly defined is in how midwives support women in established labour. Techno-rationalist approaches to labour pain emphasise its relief. Intuitive support of women in labour emanates from an anthropological reading of labour as a 'rite of passage' that includes the fundamental notion that this kind of pain can be transformative (Leap and Anderson, 2008).

This nurturing approach is almost certainly what birth companions have done over millions of years of childbirth on the planet. It is only in recent centuries that, as birth attendants have become professionalised, they have taken on technical skills which have tended to marginalise supportive, nurturing skills.

Preparation of birth partners

There is a recognition that there is a need to support fathers to support their partners during pregnancy, birth and during the transition to parenthood

(Fisher, 2007; Steen *et al.*, 2011). Yet there is evidence that approximately 60 per cent of mothers feel that their partners get little or no support during the antenatal period, with the extent of support dropping off markedly in lower social groups (NHS, 2005). *Maternity Matters* (Department of Health, 2007) recommends that high-quality maternity care should involve access to a wide range of services that work in partnership to help equip mothers and *fathers* with the skills they require to become confident and caring parents.

During pregnancy there are many opportunities for midwives to involve fathers in maternity care. No other health professional has as much routine contact with fathers as midwives do (Fisher, 2007). Many fathers in developing countries now accompany their partners at antenatal consultations, scans and parenting education. Yet men have reported high levels of stress and anxiety when their partners are pregnant (Condon *et al.*, 2004; Johnson and Baker, 2004; Rosich-Medina and Shetty, 2007).

Singh and Newburn (2003) asked men what they think of midwives and reported that most have positive opinions but highlighted the need for more holistic care for mothers and fathers. Kaila-Behm and Vehvilanen-Julkeunen (2000) found that midwives have opportunities to work closely with fathers and gain an insight into their needs. However, another study reported that most expectant fathers rely on second-hand information that is passed on by their partners (Locock and Alexander, 2006).

Approximately 50 years ago, Dick-Read (1959) said that the role of the health professional is to involve and educate the father 'with kindly-stern authority, to urge that the husband learns with his wife, the phenomena and common sense of this natural human function'. Therefore, midwives need to address this deficit and engage more with expectant fathers regardless of the birth place choice of the expectant mother. When an expectant mother opts for a homebirth, an excellent opportunity to gain access to the father is created. This opportunity should be maximised and expectant fathers should be given opportunities to be involved in antenatal preparation for the birth.

> The involvement of fathers/partners in planning and attending homebirth is encouraged as pregnancy and birth are the first major opportunities to engage fathers/partners in the appropriate care and upbringing of their children.
>
> (RCOG/RCM, 2007, p. 3)

Preparing fathers for the birth tends to lead to them being more active participants and their partners' birth experiences tend to be better (Diemer, 1997; Wockel *et al.*, 2007). Hallgren and colleagues (1999) found antenatal education to be effective in preparing fathers to take active roles at the birth.

Steen and Calvert (2007), when exploring the use of a homeopathic childbirth kit, found that when a woman's partner is well prepared and given advice and support, he is very able to take an active role in supporting his labouring partner and that both are more likely to have a positive birth experience.

A recently published book entitled *The Father's Homebirth Book* (Hazard, 2008) provides a useful resource as it explores some fathers hopes and fears around homebirth and gives valuable insight into some fathers' experiences (Figure 4.2).

Involving fathers: other benefits to the mother and baby

The home environment gives midwives an ideal opportunity to give one-to-one care and advice. Expectant fathers as well as expectant mothers are in their own familiar surroundings and more likely to feel relaxed. When women

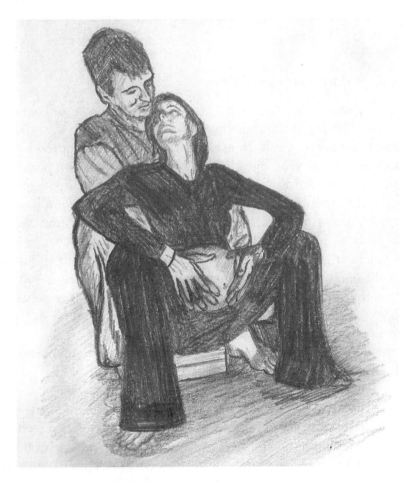

FIGURE 4.2 Man supporting his partner in labour.

opt for a homebirth, opportunities during the pregnancy for a home visit and time following the birth are available to discuss healthy lifestyle choices.

There is evidence that when the woman's partner is involved in her pregnancy, clinical outcomes for mothers and babies are improved, as are rates of smoking cessation and breast-feeding (Flouri and Buchanan, 2003; Botoroff *et al.*, 2006; British Market Research Bureau, 2007). For example, knowledge of the impact of smoking on a baby is associated with a higher chance of fathers quitting smoking (Stanton *et al.*, 2004). A father's behaviour and attitude can also influence the mother's decision to initiate and sustain breast-feeding (Schmidt and Sigman-Grant, 2000; Pollock *et al.*, 2002; Shaker *et al.*, 2004). Specific engagement with fathers can increase the number of mothers breast-feeding at six months by 70–300 per cent (Cohen *et al.*, 2002; Piscane *et al.*, 2005).

The woman's partner also has a key influence on the quality of care for the baby – both through his own contribution and through his impact on the quality of care provided by the mother (Santos Pérez *et al.*, 1998; Henwood and Proctor, 2003).

Preparing and involving children

The expectant mother and her partner may ask the midwife to help them in preparing their other children, who may be in the home whilst she is labouring and might be present for the birth itself. The use of storybooks and DVDs can help with this task (Royal College of Midwives, 2003), as can putting aside valuable family time to discuss with children what is going to happen and what they will actually see. Introducing children to another family who have experienced homebirth can be beneficial (Royal College of Midwives, 2003). This will include open discussions with the children about what happens in pregnancy, labour and birth. How much exposure to the birth children have is entirely the decision of the expectant mother and her partner. It will depend on how comfortable the couple feel with some aspects of the actual birth, such as being seminaked or worrying if the children will become distressed at watching and hearing their mother in pain.

The midwife will discuss with them some of the circumstances when it may not be appropriate for children to be present, for example when a deviation from normal occurs. There are no age limitations for the presence of children at a homebirth. If children are at school or if time out is agreed by the parents, this should be arranged ahead of time. Children should be encouraged to continue as normal and be allowed to come and go as they need (Royal College of Midwives, 2003) and may be able to participate (Figure 4.3); however, additional supervision from another family member or close friend should be

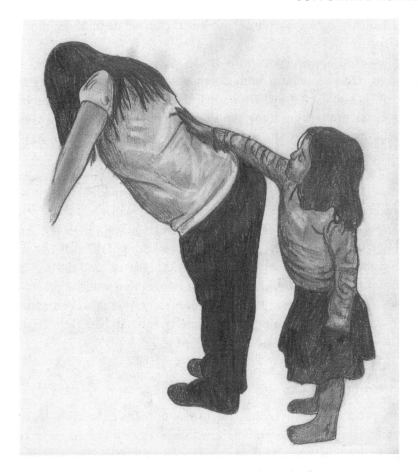

FIGURE 4.3 A child may be able to massage her mother's back.

readily available for the duration of the childbirth process. There are no rights or wrongs or ways of anticipating children's reactions to the experience so alternative arrangements should be in place if everything does not go to plan.

Homebirth care pathway

Registering for homebirth

The booking interview is one of the most important appointments for a woman during her pregnancy; not only for the opportunity to exercise choice regarding her care and antenatal screening but also to consider her place of birth. Many women assume this is not an option and that hospital birth is the norm (National Institute for Health and Clinical Excellence, 2007; BirthChoiceUK, 2009b). Exploring choice of place of birth in a positive way can influence and empower women to choose a homebirth if they have normal pregnancies and are low risk.

Midwives need appropriate skills to discuss choices with women. Asking the question 'Do you want a home or hospital birth?' will usually elicit the response of 'hospital birth' (BirthChoice UK, 2009b). Even if women do not make a decision at booking, they should be informed that this is a choice they can make at any stage of their pregnancy. It is vital that partners are involved in this decision as it is often their concerns that may influence a women's choice of place of birth (Steen *et al.*, 2011).

Once the decision to have a homebirth has been made, all health professionals who will be involved in the woman's care will need to be informed. The GP and health visitor will need to be notified as well as all the midwifery team, labour ward and supervisor of midwives. Some GPs still carry out the neonatal examination, but this is increasingly being carried out by midwives who are qualified to do so. Practising in a home environment where there is no immediate help in an emergency demands that midwives are confident and competent in all aspects of midwifery practices and have the skills to deal with emergencies when they arise (see Chapter 6).

Risk assessment

The whole process of delivering care in the homebirth setting, as with any other setting, is underpinned by the need to recognise and manage risk. It is important to look at key issues that have been identified as contributing to suboptimal care for homebirth and to ensure that systems and procedures are in place to address these to minimise risk and promote a safe homebirth service.

In the 1990s the following issues were identified as contributing to suboptimal care for homebirth (Confidential Enquiry into Stillbirth and Deaths in Infancy, 1998):

- identification and management of fetal distress;
- communication issues;
- transport issues;
- record-keeping;
- neonatal resuscitation;
- difficulty in obtaining professional support for home delivery;
- response by hospital following transfer.

To address these issues and ensure a safe homebirth service is in place it is essential to involve local multidisciplinary teams and users to underpin homebirth practices within a clinical governance framework that demonstrates commitment to supporting women in their choices (RCOG/RCM, 2007). This will promote responsible and responsive practice that is maintained by effective clinical decision-making. Maternity services must therefore:

- implement guidelines specifically for homebirth and midwifery-led care and update these regularly;
- provide staff with access to training in homebirth and obstetric skills drills, including maternal and neonatal resuscitation;
- provide training in risk management processes and operate a robust incident reporting system;
- facilitate communication between health professionals, women, their partner and families that enables continuity of care;
- ensure that midwives caring for women at home identify possible risks and plan appropriately to reduce these through their approach to care, their knowledge of local support systems and good communication with colleagues, women, their partner and their families;
- implement referral policies that recognise that, for the majority of women, pregnancy and childbirth are normal life events and that promoting choice and control over the childbirth experience can have a significant effect on children's healthy development;
- recognise that other agencies, particularly the regional ambulance service, have an integral role in the collaborative management of homebirth services and that developing a service agreement with these agencies will provide an effective transfer in service;
- consider the clinical and personal safety of the midwife practitioner at a homebirth, for example by providing minimum agreed levels of equipment.

Woman's perspective

A risk assessment needs to be performed on all women who choose a homebirth. This should include physical, emotional/psychological social and environmental risk factors. It is important to consider the woman's perceived risks as well as the risks that are considered to be a medical cause for concern. Most maternity units have standardised assessment forms which can be adapted to meet individual needs.

Risk assessment: checklist

Physical

If there are any risk factors, the woman should be offered a consultant appointment to discuss the potential risks with her. These could be existing health problems or problems which have developed during the pregnancy. The woman needs to be informed that there is a possibility that she may be advised to have a hospital birth but ultimately it is her decision.

Emotional/psychological

The risk assessment should consider the following aspects:

- How does the woman feel that she will cope at home?
- Is she emotionally prepared?
- Does she have any previous history of psychological or any other mental health problems?
- Has she had a previous traumatic birth?
- Has she had any emotional or psychological problems during this pregnancy?
- Has she considered how she will manage her labour?
- Is she anxious and showing any signs of stress?

Social and environmental

Risk areas to consider in this category include:

- Does the woman have good support and who will be with her in labour?
- Does she have any other children?
- If she does, how old are they and has she considered whether she would like them to be around during her labour and the birth itself?
- Will another family member be available to care for them?
- Has she considered the pain management options available to her?
- Is she aware of how to source pain management and also keep drugs safe in her home?
- Does her home have adequate heating and lighting?

Access and availability

Consideration of access is important. The following should be determined:

- Is there a landline phone or a good mobile phone signal?
- Could an ambulance access the property easily in an emergency? If this is difficult, ambulance control should be notified when the on-call period starts.
- How difficult is it to attend in bad weather?
- Is the property safe?

- Are there any hazards that the midwives may encounter when accessing the home? It should be noted that not all women live in a house. For example, they could live in a tent, on a boat or in a very high-rise flat.
- How long will it take for an ambulance to arrive in an emergency?
- How long will it take the midwives to get to the woman's home? This is important as the on-call midwife could live a considerable distance from the woman's home.
- Are there dogs or other animals which could pose a problem?
- What time of year is the woman expected to give birth? Weather can be problematic or there may be problems with staff shortages owing to holidays or sickness. Or there may be a large number of women due at the same time.
- It is important that there is a good relationship between the woman and her midwife and that the woman is willing to be guided by the midwife's decision if a problem arises and hospital transfer is necessary.

Equipment

Medical gases

There are variations in practice as to how the medical gases are taken to the woman's home. Some areas deliver Entonox and oxygen when an on-call midwife requests these. In other areas midwives take their own equipment and collect the gases on the way. In north Wales, fully equipped 'homebirth vans' can be accessed by the on-call midwife. Whichever method is used, the woman needs to be informed and local policies adhered to. If the gases are left at the woman's home, she needs to be aware how to store them safely and to inform her household insurance company that gases are being temporarily stored in the home.

Drugs

Drug administration and storage will be in guidance with local policies and procedures and NMC regulations (Nursing and Midwifery Council, 2007). If the midwife carries drugs she must ensure that they are stored safely. All drugs must be checked and in date. The woman must also be aware of the process for discarding any unused drugs that have been prescribed for her by the GP such as pethidine or diamorphine. All equipment must be checked and signed by the midwife stocking the homebirth bag. It is useful to have a laminated checklist for easy reference when restocking equipment. The kits should be standardised within teams. Midwives will then be confident accessing the kits in an emergency.

When to call the midwife and in an emergency

The woman and her partner should be given information on how and when to call the midwife when labour commences. They should also be told what happens in an emergency. They should be given the relevant phone numbers. It is useful to have laminated cards which can be prominently displayed when the woman is in labour in case of an emergency.

These could include information such as:

- midwife's name;
- midwife's telephone number;
- woman's gestation and expected date of delivery (EDD);
- woman's date of birth;
- how to call for help in an emergency.

If an emergency occurs and the partner has to phone for help it is easier for him to read the information off a card.

Labour/birth equipment and resources

A well-organised stocking system must be established to support homebirths. All equipment and drugs need to be adequately stocked, within their expiry date and regularly maintained, ensuring all that is needed is at hand and in working order. To promote safety of the woman and the neonate it is good practice to apply a structure and organise all equipment and drugs into separate labelled boxes or bags (Gwillim, 2009) (Table 4.2). Midwives need to become familiar with the equipment and the location of specific items so that issues of finding equipment are minimised and the focus can be on the delivery of care.

There are items and consumables that the woman and her partner will be expected to provide. The partner may need some advice on what to prepare for labour and delivery. It may be helpful if a list is prepared together with the midwife, woman and her partner. Many items will be essential and others optional. None of the items need to be purchased from new. It is important to show sensitivity to a family's financial constraints. If families are struggling financially it is helpful to anticipate the scenario and plan ahead. Many items can be shared or even donated from other families who have experienced homebirth (Royal College of Midwives, 2003).

The woman will need to know what items she needs to provide. This includes:

TABLE 4.2 Equipment and resources required for labour and homebirth

Birth bag/box

Delivery pack and instruments for suturing
Water-based vaginal lubricating jelly
Non-sterile gloves
Amnihook
Container for placenta
Selection of syringes and needles: 2 ml, 5 ml, 10 ml
Tourniquet
Alcohol wipes
Suture materials and instruments (if not contained in delivery pack)
Sanitary towels
Pinard stethoscope
Incontinence pads
Selection of blood bottles
Vacutainer set
Intravenous fluids
Sterile vaginal examination (VE) pack or materials to perform the procedure
Sterile gloves
Sonicaid to reassure mother
Sterile gauze/cotton wall balls
Anti-D antibody if woman rhesus negative
Sharps box
Rubbish bag to take items back the hospital

Drugs in separate container (drug box)

Syntometrine/Syntocinon
Local anaesthetic
Ergometrine
Vitamin K

Gases

Entonox
Oxygen

Antenatal/postnatal bag/box

Pinard stethoscope
Thermometer
Swabs for microbiology, swabs for culture
Cord clamp remover
Scissors
Sonicaid
Lancets

TABLE 4.2 (continued)

Mid-stream urine sample bottles

Torch

Tape measure

Sphygmomanometer

Plasters

Cord clamp if not in delivery pack

Baby scales that comply with Weighing Medical Regulations (2003)

Documentation/record-keeping pack

Additional recording sheets for care records

Neonatal blood spot screening cards and envelopes

Various pathology forms

Birth notification forms

Neonatal examination forms

Paper for referral letters

Partogram/established labour/birth

Postnatal exercise sheets

Envelopes

Transfer to care to health visitors documentation

Headed notepaper (factors, letters, etc.)

Emergency bag

Maternal resuscitation equipment: oxygen masks, medium concentration, pocket mask with one-way valve and various oral airways, bag–valve–mask (BVM) device (optional – as the pocket mask and oxygen is effective for basic life support) and oxygen cylinder with variable flowmeter

Neonatal resuscitation equipment: oxygen funnel, suction device, self-inflating 500-ml BVM device

Access to phone, fully charged mobile phone

Intravenous giving set and fluids (normal saline, Hartmann's solution, Gelofusion/Haemaccel)

Grey large-bore cannulae (×4)

Selection of small cannulae

Three-way tap

Plaster and i.v. sterile fixing tape

Dressing

Sterile gloves

Unsterile gloves

Label for drug additives

Pinard stethoscopes

Plastic apron

Incontinence pads and sanitary towels

Blood bottles for haemoglobin, cross-matching and forms

- a large plastic sheet or shower curtain;
- towels to dry the baby;
- a warm radiator or hot water bottle to warm baby clothes;
- tea, coffee and light refreshments for the midwives, who may be there a considerable time.

She must be informed that an area will need to be provided for resuscitation if necessary. This equipment needs to be set up on arrival at the home She should also pack a bag for her and the baby, in case of transfer to hospital.

The birth plan

Following the information-giving and risk assessment, the woman should be encouraged to make a birth plan and an individualised plan of care formulated. The birth plan will form the basis of her care pathway during labour. This needs to be discussed in partnership with her to enable her to achieve her optimum birth experience. The birth plan should be realistic and flexible and focus on the three stages of labour. Issues to be addressed include the following:

- Where does she want to labour and give birth? This may involve rearranging furniture or lighting. It should be established who will be doing this.
- Who will be with her for support?
- Who will look after any other children?
- What coping strategies will she use, for example birthing balls, music, TENS, aromatherapy, homeopathy or other alternative remedies?
- What positions can be assumed in labour and birth and how her partner can help.
- What form of pain relief is available. The woman should be taught the importance of working with the pain for the optimum outcome.
- Breathing and relaxation techniques should be taught.
- The woman should be advised that her GP will prescribe pharmacological pain relief if she requests it and she needs to be made aware of the risks and side-effects.
- If she wants a waterbirth, who will be providing the pool? A discussion should take place around the benefits and risks and she must be made aware that she may have to exit the pool at any time during the labour or birth.
- The importance of eating and drinking in labour should be discussed.
- Does she have facilities for iced or cool drinks?

- Does she want an active or physiological third stage? The risks and benefits should be explained.
- Informed consent for vitamin K to be administered must be obtained.
- Who discovers sex of the baby if not already known?
- Who will cut the cord?
- Skin-to-skin contact should be offered.
- Method of feeding discussed. If breast-feeding, enquire if she would like baby to suckle as soon as possible. If formula feeding, establish that they have sterilising equipment and formula feed.

The birth plan visit should take place at around 36 weeks' gestation, as recommended by NICE (National Institute for Health and Clinical Excellence, 2007) and, ideally, the partner should be present. In addition to formulating the birth plan, at this visit the woman will be given details of the on-call midwives, that is, who to contact and when. (There are variations in practice.) Some areas have designated homebirth teams, whereas others use community on-call or hospital based on-call midwives. The contact details should be clearly documented. It is important that any concerns are communicated to the on-call midwives and to the labour ward.

In addition, the woman's details should be circulated to the teams. This should include:

- name and address, including postcode;
- instructions on how to get to the home, and telephone number;
- the expected date of delivery and gravid status.

Midwives' skills, confidence and competencies

Many midwives on registration may not have assisted homebirths, and it is important that they are confident and competent when attending and supporting a woman to give birth at home. A midwife who lacks confidence will be unable to empower the woman to achieve a positive outcome. Mentoring and buddying with experienced midwives will enhance confidence and encourage newer midwives to promote homebirth as an option for women. Emergency skills drills should be part of mandatory training and all midwives should be competent in neonatal and maternal resuscitation.

Some maternity units, such as Maelor Hospital in north Wales, organise specific homebirth training days. This encourages evidence-based practice and the sharing of experiences. Risk meetings specific to homebirth are also a useful way of addressing adverse incidents and promotes learning in practice in a no blame culture. See homebirth case studies 4 and 7 in Chapter 8.

TABLE 4.3 Items for the expectant mother to obtain

Essential items

Protective polyurethane sheet for delivery, which needs to be large enough to protect the flooring and enable unrestricted movement by the mother: 1.5 metres by 1.5 metres is sufficient

Equipment that enables the woman to cope with pain through the stages of labour, for example paracetamol for early labour pain relief and, if required, a transcutaneous electrical nerve stimulation (TENS) machine. Some maternity units lend or hire out TENS machines

Mobility and distraction aids: pillows, large cushions, bean bags, birthing ball, duvet, flannels for hot and cold compresses, towels and a bowl

Sanitary packs (×6)

Plastic bag for rubbish

Loose clothing for mother including loose pants

Linen and blankets for cot and advice when to make it up in readiness for birth

Hot water bottle to be used for the woman for pain relief of which can be put into the neonate's cot to warm it in readiness for birth

Newborn nappies and baby clothes

Drinks and snacks for mother, partner and family

Additional items

Drinks for all attendants – if none to be provided this should be made clear so midwives can provide for themselves. They will need an area to prepare light snacks and drinks, with access to electricity for kettle

Inviting space for midwife and assistant

Aromatherapy – massage oils and implements advised and administered by a qualified practitioner

Homeopathic preparation as advised by qualified practitioner

Camera

Fan (electric or hand held)

Hand mirror

Lip balm

Music

Midwife safety

Many homebirths occur during the night, and this is an additional risk factor for midwives who have to drive to women's homes. There are several measures that midwives can take to ensure that they are remain as safe as possible:

- Obtain directions and make sure that they have the postcode and any information regarding accessibility to the home. They should take a trial run in daytime if unsure.

- Make sure that there is adequate petrol in the car and that the car is roadworthy.
- Carry a map and satnav if possible.
- Keep their mobile phone charged.
- Have a torch, shovel and blanket in the car in winter.
- Inform the labour ward when leaving home and on arrival back.
- Advise the woman in advance to keep animals out of the way.
- If the woman is high risk or the environment is unsafe, travel with another midwife.
- In adverse weather conditions, such as snow and ice, midwives should not put themselves at risk and women should be transferred to hospital by ambulance.

Conclusions

It is important that midwives actively promote normal birth practices, which will in turn assist them to support and care for women who request homebirths. To help them to do this they will need to reflect upon the importance of 'being with woman' and ways to promote normal birth practices. They will need to increase their knowledge and understanding of how anxiety and fear can have a negative impact upon childbirth. In addition, midwives need to be aware that fear of childbirth can influence women's birth place choices and they should be proactive in reducing this fear and promoting homebirth. Good preparation is the key to minimising risk and it is essential to address safety issues and have the knowledge of procedures and systems in place to support women requesting a homebirth.

It is vitally important for midwives to involve women's partners or family members who will be with her during labour and birth, so that they feel confident in this role.

References

Albers, L. (1999) The duration of labour in healthy women. *Journal of Perinatology*, 19, 114–19.

Alehagen, S., Wijma, B., Lundberg, U. and Wijma, K. (2005) Fear, pain and stress hormones during childbirth. *Journal of Psychosomatic Obstetrics and Gynaecology*, 26, 153–65.

American Medical Association. (2008) Resolution on home deliveries (http://www.ama-assn.org/ama1/pub/upload/mm/471/205.doc).

Anon. (2011) Editorial. *American Journal of Obstetrics and Gynecology*, 204(4), pe20 (http://www.ajog.org/issues?issue_key=S0002-9378(11)X000300; accessed 20 May 2011).

American College of Obstetricians and Gynecologists (2008) Statement on Home Births (http://www.acog.org/from_home/publications/press_releases/nr02-06-08-2.cfm).

Australian Institute of Health and Welfare (2003) *Rural, Regional and Remote Health: A Study on Mortality*. Cat. no. PHE 45; rural health series no. 2. Canberra: Australian Institute of Health and Welfare.

Bastick, T. (1982) *Intuition: How We Think and Act*. New York: John Wiley & Sons.

BirthChoiceUK (2009a) Home Birth Rates (http://www.birthchoiceuk.com/BirthChoiceUKFrame. htm?http://www.birthchoiceuk.com/HomeBirthRates.htm; accessed 8 March 2011).

BirthChoiceUK (2009b) Index of National Maternity Statistics (http://www.birthchoiceuk.com/ Professionals/Frame.htm; accessed 8 March 2011).

Bottorff, J.L., Oliffe, J., Kalaw, C., Carey, J. and Mroz, L. (2006) Men's constructions of smoking in the context of women's tobacco reduction during pregnancy and postpartum. *Social Science and Medicine*, 62, 3096–108.

Boucher, B., Bennett, C., McFarlin, B. and Freeze, R. (2009) Staying home to give birth: why women in the United States choose home birth. *Journal of Midwifery and Women's Health*, 54(2), 119–26.

British Market Research Bureau (2007) *Infant Feeding Survey 2005*. A survey conducted on behalf of the Information Centre for Health and Social Care and the UK Health Departments. Southport: The Information Centre.

Brockington, I. (1998) *Motherhood and Mental Health*. Oxford: Oxford University Press.

Buckley, S.J. (2005) *Gentle Birth, Gentle Mothering*. Brisbane: One Moon Press.

Cohen, R., Lange, L. and Slusser, W. (2002) A description of a male-focused breastfeeding promotion corporate lactation programme. *Journal of Human Lactation*, 18, 61–5.

Condon, J.T., Boyce, P. and Corkindale, C.J. (2004) The first-time father's study: a prospective study of the mental health and wellbeing of men during the transition to parenthood. *Australian and New Zealand Journal of Psychiatry*, 38, 56–64.

Confidential Enquiry into Stillbirth and Deaths in Infancy (1998) 5th Annual Report. London: Maternal and Child Health Research Consortium, London.

Cooper, T. and Clarke, P. (2008) Freebirthing: home alone – a concerning trend. *Midwives*, 11(3), 34–5.

Davies, L. (2004) 'Allowed' shouldn't be allowed! *MIDIRS Midwifery Digest*, 14, 151–6.

Davis-Floyd, R. (2001) The technocratic, humanistic and holistic paradigms of childbirth. *International Journal of Gynaecology and Obstetrics*, 75, S5–23.

Department of Health (2004) *National Service Framework for Children, Young People and Maternity Services*. London: Department of Health.

Department of Health (2007) *Maternity Matters: Choice, Access and Continuity of Care in a Safe Service*. London: HMSO.

Department of Health (2010) *Maternity and Early Years: Making a Good Start to Family Life*. London: HMSO.

Devane, D., Brennan, M., Begley, C., Clarke, M., Walsh, D., Sandall, J., Ryan, P., Revill, P. and Normand, C. (2010) A systematic review, meta-analysis, meta-synthesis and economic analysis of midwife-led models of care. London: Royal College of Midwives (http://www. rcm.org.uk/college/campaigns-events/value-of-the-midwife/; accessed 23 May 2011).

Dick-Read, G. (1959) *Childbirth without Fear*, 4th edn. London: Heinemann Medical Books.

Dick-Read, G. (2004) *Childbirth without Fear: The Principles and Practice of Natural Childbirth* (reissued edition). London: Pinter & Martin.

Diemer, G. (1997) Expectant fathers: influence of perinatal education on coping, stress, and spousal relations. *Research in Nursing and Health*, 20, 281–93.

Dietsch, E., Shackleton, P., Davies, C., Alston, M. and McLeod, M. (2010) 'Mind you, there's no anaesthetist on the road': women's experiences of labouring en route. *Rural and Remote Health*, 10 (online), 1371 (http://www.rrh.org.au; accessed 4 May 2010).

Emerson, W.R. (1998) Birth trauma: the psychological effects of obstetrical interventions. *Journal of Prenatal, Perinatal Psychology & Health*, 13(1), 11–44.

Ekin, M., Keirse, M., Neilson, J., Crowther, C., Duley, L., Hodnett, E. and Hofmeyr, J. (2000) *Guide to Effective Care in Pregnancy and Childbirth*, 3rd edn. Oxford: Oxford Medical Publications.

European Court of Human Rights (2010) Legal uncertainty prevented mother from giving birth at home, Press release no. 962, issued by the Registrar of the Court, Strasbourg, 14

December 2010 (http://cmiskp.echr.coe.int/tkp197/portal.asp?sessionId=68904503&skin=hudoc-pr-en&action=request; accessed 31 March 2011).

Fisher, D (2007) Including New Fathers. A Guide for Maternity Professionals (http://www.fathersdirect.com).

Fisher, D. (2009) Should men be at the birth of babies? What I said in the debate with Michel Odent. Duncan Fisher. The blog of Duncan Fisher OBE, home entrepreneur (http://www.duncanfisher.com/index.php/2009/11/27/should-men-be-at-the-birth-of-babies-what-i-said-in-the-debate-with-michel-odent/; accessed 3 March 2011).

Flouri, E. and Buchanan, A. (2003) What predicts fathers' involvement with their children? A prospective study of intact families. *British Journal of Developmental Psychology*, 21, 81–97.

Frye, A. (2004) Anatomy and physiology of uterine changes during late pregnancy and labor. In *Holistic Midwifery: A Comprehensive Textbook for Midwives in Homebirth Practice. Vol. II: Care of the Mother and Baby from the Onset of Labor through the First Hours after Birth*. Oregon: Labrys Press, pp. 256–2.

Gaskin, I.M. (2008) *Ina May's Guide to Childbirth*. London: Vermilion.

Gwillim, J. (2009) Home birth. In Chapman, V. and Charles, C. (eds.) *The Midwife's Labour and Birth Handbook*, 2nd edn. Oxford: Wiley-Blackwell.

Gyte, G., Dodwell, M., Newburn, M., Sandall, J., MacFarlane, A. and Bexley, S. (2010) Findings of a meta-analysis can not be relied on. *BMJ*, 341, c4033.

Hancock, H. (2007) Low birth weight in Aboriginal babies – a need for rethinking Aboriginal women's pregnancies and birthing. *Women and Birth*, 20(2), 77–80.

Hallgren, A., Kihlgren, M., Forslin, L. and Norberg, A. (1999) Swedish fathers' involvement in and experiences of childbirth preparation and childbirth. *Midwifery*, 15, 6–15.

Hazard, L. (2008) *The Father's Homebirth Book*. London: Pinter & Martin.

Henwood, K. and Proctor, J. (2003) The 'good father': reading men's accounts of paternal involvement during the transition to first-time fatherhood. *British Journal of Social Psychology*, 42, 337–55.

Hill, A. (2010) Hungary: Midwife Agnes Gereb taken to court for championing home births. *The Guardian*, 22 October 2010 (http://www.guardian.co.uk/world/2010/oct/22/hungary-midwife-agnes-gereb-home-birth).

Hodnett, E.D., Downe, S., Walsh, D. and Weston, J. (2010) Alternative versus conventional institutional settings for birth. *Cochrane Database of Systematic Reviews*, Issue 9, article no. CD000012 (DOI 10.1002/14651858.CD000012.pub3).

Hodnett, E.D., Gates, S., Hofmeyr, G.J., Sakala, C. and Weston, J. (2011) Continuous support for women during childbirth. *Cochrane Database of Systematic Reviews*, Issue 2, article no. CD003766 (DOI 10.1002/14651858.CD003766.pub3).

Hunt, Lord (2000) quoted in Lords Hansard text, House of Lords, Maternity Services, 20 December 2000: Column 73 (http://www.publications.parliament.uk/pa/ld200001/ldhansrd/vo001220/text/01220-01.htm#01220-01_head; accessed 28 February 2011).

Hunter, B. (2005) The need for change – the midwives' perspective. *MIDIRS Midwifery Digest*, 15(4), Suppl. 2, s2–25.

Independent Midwives UK (2011) Health Professionals: Who We Are (http://www.independentmidwives.org.uk/?node=608; accessed 31 March 2011).

International Confederation of Midwives (2008) *Keeping Birth Normal*. Position Statement. The Hague: International Confederation of Midwives.

Johnson, M.P. and Baker, S.R. (2004) Implications of coping repertoire as predictors of men's stress, anxiety and depression following pregnancy, childbirth and miscarriage: a longitudinal study. *Journal of Psychosomatic Obstetrics and Gynaecology*, 25, 87–98.

de Jonge, A., van der Goes, B., Ravelli, A., Amelink-Verberg, M., Mol, B., Nijhuis, J., Bennebroek Gravenhorst, J. and Buitendijk, S. (2009) Perinatal mortality and morbidity in a nationwide cohort of 529688 low-risk planned home and hospital births. *BJOG* (DOI: 10.1111/j.1471-0528.2009.02175x).

Kaila-Behm, A. and Vehvilainen-Julkunen, K. (2000) Ways of being a father: how first-time fathers and public health nurses perceive men as fathers. *International Journal of Nursing Studies*, 37, 199–205.

King James Version (2010) 'Book of Genesis 16. . . in *The Bible* (http://www.blueletterbible.org/Bible.cfm?b=Gen&c+35RV=16&E=KJV#16; last accessed 25 May 2010).

Kitzinger. S. (2000) Introduction: searching questions about birth. In *Rediscovering Birth*. London: Little Brown & Co., p. 11.

Kitzinger, S. (2002) *Birth Your Way: Choosing Birth at Home or in a Birth Centre*. New York: Dorling Kindersley.

Leap, N. and Anderson, P. (2008) The role of pain in normal birth and the empowerment of women. In Downe, S. (ed.) *Normal Childbirth: Evidence and Debate,* 2nd edn. London: Churchill Livingstone.

Locock, L. and Alexander, J (2005) 'Just a bystander?' Men's place in the process of fetal screening and diagnosis. *Social Science and Medicine*, 62, 1349–59.

Melender, H. (2002) Experiences of fears associated with pregnancy and childbirth: a study of 329 women. *Birth*, 27(3), 101–11.

Murphy, D.J., Pope, C., Frost, J. and Liebling, R. (2003) Women's views on the impact of operative delivery in the second stage of labour: qualitative interview study. *BMJ*, 327, 1132.

NHS Quality Improvement Scotland (2009) *Pathways for Maternity Care.* (http://www.nhshealthquality.org/nhsqis/files/Final%20KCND%20pathway[1].pdf; accessed 5 May 2010).

NHS Wales (2006) All Wales Clinical Pathway for Normal Labour. (http://www.wales.nhs.uk/sites3/home.cfm?orgid=327; accessed 28 February 2011).

Nursing and Midwifery Council (NMC) (2007) *Standards for Medicines Management*. London: NMC.

Nolan, M.L. (2011) Free birth: the end of the choice continuum. In *Homebirth: The Politics of Difficult Choices*. Abingdon: Routledge.

National Perinatal Epidemiology Unit (2010) Birth Place in England Research Programme. Oxford: National Perinatal Epidemiology Unit (http://www.npeu.ox.ac.uk/birthplace; accessed 5 May 2010).

NHS (2005) *Maternity Services Quantitative Research*. Prepared by TNS System Three for Katie Hawkins. London: Department of Health.

National Institute for Health and Clinical Excellence (2007) *Intrapartum Care*. Clinical Guideline 55. London: National Institute for Health and Clinical Excellence.

NHS Knowledge (2009) Homebirth 'safe as in hospital'. Health News, NHS Choices Information (http://www.nhs.uk/news/2009/04April/Pages/HomeBirthSafe.aspx; accessed 14 August 2011).

Nursing and Midwifery Council (2004) *Code of Professional Standards for Conduct, Performance and Ethics*. London: Nursing and Midwifery Council.

Nursing and Midwifery Council (2007) *Standards for Medicines Management*. London: Nursing and Midwifery Council.

O'Connell, S., Williams, B. and Richley, A. (2011) Feeling right at home: homebirth. *RCM Midwives Journal*, 2, 28–9.

Ólafsdóttir, Ó.Á. (2010) The Art and Science of Midwifery: At the Side of the Woman? (http://www.barnmorskeforbundet.se/images/content/documents/Olof_Asta_Olofsdottir_Presentation_OAO_The_Art_and_Science_of_Midwifery_-_At_the_Side_of_the_Woman.pdf; accessed 31 March 2011).

Olsen, O. and Jewell, D. (1998) Home versus hospital birth. *Cochrane Database of Systematic Reviews*, Issue 3, article no. CD000352 (DOI: 10.1002/14651858.CD000352).

Piscane A., Continisio G.I., Aldinucci M., D'Amora S. and Continisio, P. (2005) A controlled trial of the father's role in breastfeeding promotion. *Pediatrics*, 116, 494–8.

Pollock, C.A., Bustamante-Forest, R. and Giarratano, G. (2002). Men of diverse cultures: knowledge and attitudes about breastfeeding. *Journal of Obstetric, Gynaecologic and Neonatal Nursing*, 31, 673–9.

RANZCOG (2009) *Home Birth: College Statement.* Melbourne: RANZCOG.

Royal College of Midwives (2000) *Vision 2000 Policy Document.* London: Royal College of Midwives.

Royal College of Midwives (2003) *Home Birth Handbook. Vol. 2: Practising Home Birth.* London: Royal College of Midwives.

Royal College of Midwives (2005) Campaign for Normal Birth (http://www.rcmnormalbirth. org.uk/; accessed 14 August 2011).

RCOG/RCM (2007) Joint Statement Number 2. *Home Births.* London: RCOG/RCM.

Rosich-Medina, A. and Shetty, A. (2007) Paternal experiences of pregnancy and labour. *British Journal of Midwifery*, 15(2), 66–74.

Sandall, J. (2004) Promoting normal birth: weighing the evidence. In Downe, S. (ed.) *Normal Childbirth: Evidence and Debate.* Oxford: Churchill Livingstone, pp. 161–71.

Santos Pérez, M., Lerma Soriano, A. and Ruiz Plaza, J.M. (1998) Fathers' experiences during their wives' pregnancy [in Spanish]. *Rev Enfem*, 21, 18–19.

Schmidt, M.M. and Sigman-Grant, M. (2000) Perspectives of low-income fathers' support of breastfeeding: an exploratory study. *Journal of Nutrition Education*, 32(2), 31–7.

Scottish Executive Health Department (2001) *A Framework for Maternity Services in Scotland.* Edinburgh: Scottish Executive Health Department.

Scottish Executive Health Department (2002) *Report of the Expert Group on Acute Maternity Services.* Edinburgh: Scottish Executive Health Department (http://www.scotland.gov.uk/ Resource/Doc/47021/0013918.pdf; accessed 5 May 2010).

Shaker, I., Scott, J.A. and Reid, M. (2004) Infant feeding attitudes of expectant parents: breast-feeding and formula feeding. *Journal of Advanced Nursing*, 45, 260–8.

Simpkin, P. (1991) Just another day in a woman's life: women's long-term perceptions of their birth experience. Part 1. *Birth*, 18, 203–10.

Singh, D. and Newburn, M. (2003) What men think of midwives. *RCM Midwives Journal*, 6(2), 70–4.

Sofia News Agency (2011) Homebirth in Sofia comes to a fatal end (http://www.thebulgarian-news.com/view_news.php?id=128086; accessed 27 May 2011).

Stanton, W.R., Lowe, J.B., Moffatt, J.J., and Del Marr, C. (2004) Randomized controlled trial of smoking cessation intervention directed at men whose partners are pregnant. *Preventive Medicine*, 38, 6–9.

Steen, M. and Calvert, J, (2007) Self-administered homeopathy. 2. A follow up study. *British Journal of Midwifery*, 15, 359–65.

Steen, M. and Walsh, D. (2007) Making normal birth a reality. *Revista da Associacao Portuguesa dos Enfermeiros Obstetras, Dia Internacional do Enfermeiro de Sauda Materna e Obstetrica*, 8, 15–19.

Steen, M., Downe, S. and Sapsford, N. (2010) A meta-synthesis of father's involvement in mater-nity care. First International Doctoral Midwifery Research Society Conference, University of Ulster, Northern Ireland.

Steen, M., Downe, S., Bamford, N. and Edozien, L. (2011) Not-patient and not-visitor: a meta-synthesis of fathers' encounters with pregnancy, birth and maternity care. *Midwifery* (DOI 10.1016/j.midw.2011.06).

Stephens, L. (2005) Worrying truth behind homebirth figures. *British Journal of Midwifery*, 13(1), 4–5.

Tucker, L. (2003) Fear factors: everyone reacts to fear differently. Scientists are beginning to understand why. *Science World*, 7 February, 14–15.

van Wagner, V., Epoo, B., Nastapoka, J. and Harney, E. (2007) Reclaiming birth, health and community: midwifery in the Inuit villages of Nunavik, Canada. *Journal of Midwifery and Women's Health*, 52, 384–91.

Wax, J.R., Lucas, F.L., Lamont, M., Pinette, M.G., Cartin, A. and Blackstone, J. (2010) Maternal and newborn outcomes in *planned home* birth vs *planned* hospital births: a metaanalysis. *American Journal of Obstetrics and Gynecology*, 203(3) (DOI 10.1016/j.ajog.2010.05.028).

Walsh, D. and Newburn, M. (2002) Towards a social model of childbirth. Part 1. *British Journal of Midwifery*, 10, 476–81.

Walsh, D. and Steen, M. (2007) The role of the midwife: time a review. *Midwives Journal*, 10, 320–3.

Weighing Medical Regulations (2003) Directive for Non Automatic Scales in Medicine Number 90/384/EEC, Medical Device Directive 93/42/EEC (http://www.scalesexpress.com/media/uploads/medreg2003.pdf; accessed 14 August 2011).

Wockel, A., Schafer, E., Beggel, A. and Abou-Dakn, M (2007) Getting ready for birth: impending fatherhood. *British Journal of Midwifery*, 15, 344–8.

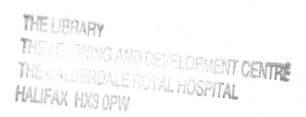

Appendix 4.1: All Wales Clinical Pathway for Normal Labour

Your Pathway Through Labour

	Prior to the onset of labour	Very early labour	Active labour - 1st stage
Expected length		Can last several days	1st baby - 6-20 hours. 2nd baby onwards - 2-10 hours
Contractions	Painless practice or "Braxton Hicks" contractions are common	Contractions feel uncomfortable but are not yet regular	Contractions are coming regularly about every 5 mins (or more frequently) and lasting 20-60 seconds
Meals	Normal, eat as usual	Small, light meals containing carbohydrates prepare the body well	Lots of fluids help, you may not feel like eating much
Monitoring	You should expect to feel at least 10 movements everyday	Keep an eye on the baby's movements at least 10 per day	The midwife will listen to the baby's heartbeat every 15 minutes, your blood pressure and temperature will be taken every 4 hours and your pulse every 30 minutes
Activity		A walk or stretching can help you relax	Remaining upright and active can mean less need for pain relief and a shorter 1st stage of labour
Support	You should be thinking about who you would like to be your birthing partners, ensure you have a contact number for your community midwife or the labour ward	You may not want to be on your own, a birth partner can hold you, rub your back and be reassuring	You are advised to contact a midwife at this stage. A midwife will care for you throughout labour
Vaginal loss	Pregnancy often increases the amount of clear vaginal discharge	You may pass a "show", the plug of mucus is released from your cervix, it can be streaked with blood. Your waters may break	The midwife will monitor the vaginal loss, your "waters" may break
Cervical Dilatation	Your cervix is closed and about 2cms in thickness	The cervix thins out	The cervix gradually dilates up to about 10 cms. This is called fully dilated.
Pain relief		Bathing, mobilising, a Tens machine, massage, relaxing music and Paracetamol (no more than 8 in 24 hours) can really help	Being active and having a bath/ shower can help & have no side effects. Pain killing drugs are available, your midwife will discuss them
How you may feel	Expectant, excited, uncertain and anxious	Excited but pace yourself, get as much rest as possible	At the end of the 1st stage, you might become a bit "tetchy" and feel you cannot cope. This is a good sign - you are nearly there.

Your Pathway Through Labour

All Wales Clinical Pathway for Normal Labour

Midwives and other members of your health care team have developed a plan of care which we anticipate you will receive. This pathway leaflet tells you about the likely pattern of care during your labour. It will help you to see what is expected to happen at any particular time.

This pathway has been developed by the health care professionals who are responsible for your care whilst you are in labour. Do not worry if you do not exactly follow the pathway; you are an individual and your labour may vary. Your plan is tailored especially to suit you.

If you have any questions regarding the normal labour pathway or the care you receive do not hesitate to ask your midwife.

Guilbert UK 04/03 LF2

	Active labour - 2nd Stage	Active labour - 3rd Stage	After the Birth
Expected length	1st baby - 1-2 hours 2nd baby onwards - 10 mins - 1 hour	20 mins - 1 hour or 5-15 mins with an injection	
Contractions	Contractions are very strong and close together with strong urges to push down	You may feel a strong urge to push your placenta out	"After pains" may make your tummy tender
Meals	Sips of fluid can help your mouth from drying out		Tea and toast has never tasted so good!
Monitoring	The midwife will listen to the baby's heartbeat every 5 minutes		Your temperature, pulse and blood pressure will be taken. The baby will be weighed and its temperature taken
Activity	Movement and changing position can help	Being upright can help your body expel the placenta	You have earned a good rest!
Support	Your midwife and birth partner's will encourage you with your pushing		The midwife will leave only when you are happy to be left
Vaginal loss	Your waters may break, the midwife will monitor the vaginal loss	A small gush of blood is usually passed before the placenta comes out	The vaginal loss can be like a heavy period for a few days
Cervical dilatation	The cervix is fully dilated		The cervix closes after the placenta and membranes are delivered
Pain relief			If you need stitches, local anaesthetic will be used to take away the discomfort
How you may feel	Very focused requiring all your efforts	An enormous relief, you will be holding your baby for this part	Very tired but totally fulfilled - congratulations

Appendix 4.2: Ternovsky v. Hungary

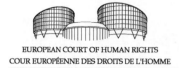

EUROPEAN COURT OF HUMAN RIGHTS
COUR EUROPÉENNE DES DROITS DE L'HOMME

Press Release
issued by the Registrar of the Court

no. 962
14.12.2010

Legal uncertainty prevented mother from giving birth at home

In today's Chamber judgment in the case Ternovszky v. Hungary (application no. 67545/09), which is not final[1], the European Court of Human Rights held, by a majority, that there had been:

A violation of Article 8 (right to respect for private and family life) of the European Convention on Human Rights

Principal facts

The applicant, Anna Ternovszky, is a Hungarian national who was born in 1979 and lives in Budapest. She was pregnant when she lodged her application with the Court.

She intended to give birth at her home, rather than in a hospital or a birth home, but alleged she had not been able to do so because health professionals were effectively dissuaded by law[2] from assisting her as they risked being convicted. It appeared that at least one such prosecution had taken place in recent years.

Complaints, procedure and composition of the Court

Relying, in particular, on Article 8 (right to respect for private and family life), the applicant alleged that the fact that she had not been able to benefit from adequate professional assistance for a home birth in view of the relevant Hungarian legislation – and as opposed to those wishing to give birth in a health institution – had amounted to discrimination in the enjoyment of her right to respect for her private life.

The application was lodged with the European Court of Human Rights on 15 December 2009.

Judgment was given by a Chamber of seven, composed as follows:

Françoise **Tulkens** (Belgium), *President*,
Danutė **Jočienė** (Lithuania),
Dragoljub **Popović** (Serbia),
András **Sajó** (Hungary),
Nona **Tsotsoria** (Georgia),
Kristina **Pardalos** (San Marino),
Guido **Raimondi** (Italy), *Judges*,

---

1 Under Articles 43 and 44 of the Convention, this Chamber judgment is not final. During the three-month period following its delivery, any party may request that the case be referred to the Grand Chamber of the Court. If such a request is made, a panel of five judges considers whether the case deserves further examination. In that event, the Grand Chamber will hear the case and deliver a final judgment. If the referral request is refused, the Chamber judgment will become final on that day.

Once a judgment becomes final, it is transmitted to the Committee of Ministers of the Council of Europe for supervision of its execution. Further information about the execution process can be found here: www.coe.int/t/dghl/monitoring/execution

2 section 101(2) of Government Decree no. 218/1999

Appendix 4.3: Royal College of Midwives press release, 23 November 2010

Royal College of Midwives calls for release of imprisoned Hungarian midwife

Commenting on the imprisonment of Hungarian midwife Agnes Gereb, Cathy Warwick, General Secretary of the Royal College of Midwives (RCM), said: 'The RCM joins professional colleagues as well as other groups from across the UK, Europe and indeed the rest of the world in registering our very strong condemnation of the treatment of Agnes Gereb. We would like to call both for the release of Dr Gereb and for the introduction of legislation in Hungary which would allow midwives to perform out of hospital births.

'Agnes Gereb is a woman who has been attempting to work in the interests of women. Her treatment at the hands of the authorities is disproportionate and inhumane. She has been arrested, imprisoned and mistreated. It is grossly unjust that any woman should be treated in such a way – shackled and handcuffed and unable to see her family for more than an absolutely minimal time over a period of forty four days. The RCM along with our sister organisation the Hungarian Midwives Association calls for her release and fair treatment.

'In addition the RCM believes it is every woman's right to choose where and how they will give birth to their baby. European-wide regulation should make it legal for midwives to work in any place that women choose to give birth. Women are aware that there is strong evidence to support out of hospital birth and in making such a choice they should not be denied the attendance of a registered midwife. The RCM calls on the Hungarian authorities to urgently address this issue.'

Chapter 5   **Caring for women during a homebirth**

Kim Gibbon and Mary Steen

Introduction

This chapter will specifically focus on preparing and caring for women during a homebirth. It will cover the care needed during early and established labour. A revision of the physiology of childbirth and mechanisms of labour is included to enable midwives to reflect on these processes to assist them to care and support women who choose a homebirth. Finally, guidance for care of the mother and baby following the birth will be discussed, and this brings the chapter to close.

The childbirth process

The birth begins when labour contractions start becoming frequent, intense and of sufficient duration to cause the cervix to open. The woman may have been experiencing Braxton Hicks contractions, which will have softened her cervix, and the hormone relaxin will have prepared the pelvic ligaments to stretch (Steen, 2011). She may have noticed that the operculum has been dislodged, which indicates that labour and birth will occur soon. She has chosen to give birth at home in her familiar surroundings and she alerts her midwife or the delivery suite that labour is commencing. She is focused and prepared for childbirth.

She knows the signs and stages of labour:

- show(s), spontaneous rupture of membranes, regular contractions;
- latent phase (early);
- stages of labour (established);
  - first stage (including a transitional phase)
  - second stage (the birth)
  - third stage (delivery of placenta and membranes).

Whether birth is difficult or easy, painful or pain free, long drawn out or brief, it need not be a medical event.

(Kitzinger, 2002, p. 7)

Physiology of labour

This section covers a revision of the physiology of childbirth, so a midwife can reflect on the process to assist her to give care and support to a woman giving birth at home.

Hormonal control

The hormonal control of labour and birth is a complex and finely tuned system which enables a woman to give birth safely (Russell, 2008). Labour and birth are primarily influenced by oxytocin, endorphins and enkephalins, the catecholamines (adrenaline and noradrenaline) and prolactin (Buckley, 2004). During labour and birth, the limbic system of the brain plays an important role. Endorphins and enkephalins are released to provide the woman with some naturally induced pain relief. In addition, the pressure of the fetus against the cervix and pelvic floor triggers the release of oxytocin and stimulates labour contractions (Russell, 2008). Therefore, it is advantageous for women to adopt an upright position during labour. Oxytocin is released from the pituitary gland and assists in the effacement and dilation of the cervix. It helps the baby to descend and negotiate the birth canal. It also assists the woman to birth her placenta, and controls bleeding. Human beings produce adrenaline (the fight or flight hormone) as a protective mechanism to survive (Cannon, 1915). Women who feel frightened and unsafe during labour will produce more adrenaline. High levels of adrenaline can slow or even stop labour (Gaskin, 2008). In human evolution, this protective mechanism assisted birthing women to move on and find a place of safety. Environmental factors continue to play an important role during labour and birth. A calm, relaxing environment helps the hormones associated with labour and birth to work in harmony and women to progress as nature planned. This is one of the reasons why the woman's home is viewed as an optimal birthing environment where normal birth is more likely to occur (Russell, 2008).

Uterine muscles

There are three types of muscle fibres in the uterus that play a part during labour and birth (Frye, 2004; Vance, 2009; Dick-Read, 2004):

- outer layer – longitudinal muscle fibres;
- middle layer – circular muscle fibres;
- inner layer – spiral muscles fibres (criss-cross).

Longitudinal muscle fibres

Longitudinal muscle fibres extend from the cervix anteriorly over the fundus of the uterus to the cervix posteriorly and play a very active role during a contraction. These fibres shorten in labour when the uterus contracts and retracts. They pull up and open the cervix during the first stage of labour. This is known as the thinning out (effacing) of the cervix and dilatation of the os uteri. During a contraction, the presenting part, usually the baby's head, is pushed down towards the cervix to assist this process and thereby facilitate the descent and expulsion of the baby, placenta and membranes.

Circular muscles

Circular muscles occur mainly in the cornua (body of uterus) and around the cervix. These fibres hold the cervix closed by resisting the longitudinal muscles but gradually give way and thin out to allow the cervix to dilate fully and be taken up and form part of the lower uterine segment so that the baby can descend through the birth canal.

Spiral muscles

The spiral (criss-cross) muscles are interwined with blood vessels that supply the uterus with oxygen and nutrients and remove waste products. These muscles are affected by the sympathetic nervous system, heart rate, respirations, blood pressure, sweat, liver function and blood sugar. When a woman is anxious and fearful, these muscles will contract and resist very strongly against the action of the longitudinal muscles. This can delay the progress of labour and can cause considerable pain. These fibres are thickest in the upper part of the uterus, where the placenta usually attaches itself during early pregnancy. They act as natural ligatures to the blood vessels when the placenta separates from the uterine wall during the third stage of labour to control bleeding.

Mechanism of labour

During evolution the human race evolved from walking on all fours to walking upright, and this involved changes to the spine and pelvis. The spine became curved and the pelvis tilted, which gave a curve to the birth canal, and during birth a baby has to negotiate this curve (the curve of Carus) and undertake rotational manoeuvres known as the 'mechanism of labour' or 'cardinal movements of birth' (Frye, 2004; Royal College of Midwives, 2005). These manoeuvres comprise:

1. flexion of the head;
2. descent;
3. engagement;
4. internal rotation of the head;

5. extension of the neck just below the occiput;
6. restitution;
7. external rotation.

A mother's pelvic floor muscles play an important role in helping her baby's head to rotate and move through her birth canal. In first-time mothers a baby's head usually descends into their pelvic inlet in a transverse diameter whereas in second-time mothers the baby's head often sits at the brim of the pelvis and will descend and enter when labour commences. During established labour a baby's head will rotate and leave the pelvic outlet through the anteroposterior diameter, which is then the largest diameter (Figure 5.1).

For the 'mechanism of labour' to progress normally, a baby must be lying longitudinally and with the head as the presenting part (as is the case in 96 per cent of births). The head is normally flexed and enters the mother's pelvic brim in the right occipitolateral (ROL), left occipitolateral (LOL), right occip-itoanterior (ROA) or left occipitoanterior (LOA) position (Frye, 2004). When the mother's uterus contracts during labour, the muscles in the upper segment of her uterus will retract and become shorter and thicker. An upwards pull

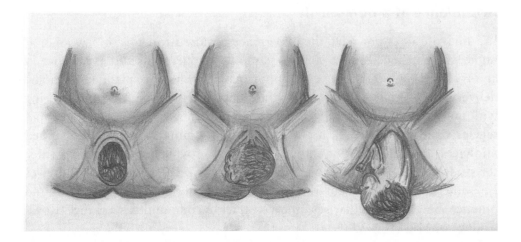

FIGURE 5.1 Baby's head rotating. Left: crowning. When the baby's head is fully visible, this is known as 'crowning'. As the head presses down on the pelvic floor it creates an urge to push or 'bear down'. Middle: head delivery. As the womb continues to contract, and the mother begins to push, the baby's head will be delivered, little by little. If the cord is around the baby's neck or body, the midwife will unravel it as the baby is born. Right: birth of the baby. Next the baby's body will be delivered, usually fairly quickly. The midwife may turn the baby slightly to help the baby's shoulders negotiate the birth canal with the next contraction.

on the lower segment of her uterus then occurs and stretches and thins this part and helps her cervix to dilate. Also, owing to the reduced capacity in her upper uterus, her baby is forced downwards, putting pressure upon her cervix to open (Figure 5.2). The cervix is taken up and becomes part of the lower segment of her uterus. When this occurs the mother is entering the second stage of labour and the baby's head and shoulders will rotate, enabling the baby to descend through her pelvis and be born.

As this is happening, the woman will feel the urge to bear down and push. A midwife will help her to remain focused, feel for a contraction and encourage her to push when she feels the urge. This will come naturally when she has a contraction but she needs to work with her body's instincts and not panic (Steen, 2011). She should adopt the position she find most comfortable and easy to give birth (Royal College of Midwives, 2006). Some mothers will make noises when bearing down whilst others will breathe deeply and quietly when doing this; it's about whatever she finds helpful and what works for her. Pushing her baby out into the world takes a huge amount of effort and energy, she may need to be reminded that she has the ability and is very capable of doing this.

Attendance at a homebirth

If a midwife does not have the experience required to care for a woman at home, she will need to take steps to gain knowledge, skills and experience in an organised way so that she can support women who have planned for home delivery. Inexperienced midwives would benefit from a period of mentoring with midwives who are highly experienced in homebirth. Homebirth competencies should be included in preceptorship programmes for newly qualified midwives, and consideration should be given to proving homebirth experience for student midwives. A period of mentorship or preceptorship for midwives encountering homebirth for the first time not only enhances safety around practice but also familiarises midwives with community working (Royal College of Midwives, 2006).

Regular attendance at homebirth study days should form part of mandatory clinical updating programmes. All midwives, not just those who practise in the community, need to keep their skills and emergency drills up to date, ensuring that they are well practised in the manoeuvres for delivering babies who are breech presentation or have shoulder dystocia, and competent in the management of postpartum haemorrhage and resuscitation of adults and neonates (see Chapter 6). Midwives must be able to cannulate and suture proficiently. Trusts should provide in-house training for midwives before they work in the community. This training should include conflict resolution and educating

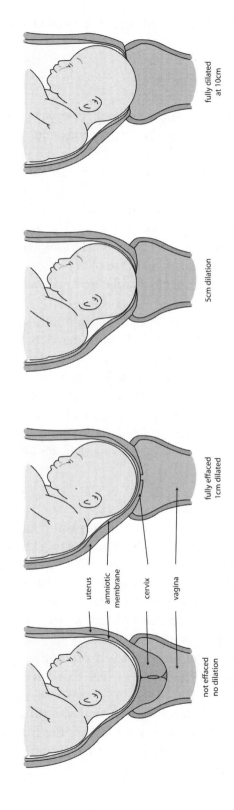

Figure 5.2 Cervix opening. Reproduced under the Creative Commons agreement. Source: Fred the Oyster.

midwives about the practicalities of using break away techniques (Heath and Safety Executive, 2009).

Working with a doula

If a woman chooses to employ a doula then it is important that midwife and doula are able to work together to the woman's benefit. A doula is a woman who is experienced in childbirth and can provide physical, emotional and informational support (Simkin, 2008). She may bring a holistic perspective (Salt, 2003), raising approaches or ways of thinking about childbirth that the midwife would not in the normal course of events consider to be critical. In addition, a doula can 'act as [the woman's] . . . advocate and constant companion. However, they cannot challenge medical or midwifery advice given to the woman or persuade her against a course of action or treatment suggested by the medical team' (for further information go to www.britishdoulas.co.uk/what-is-a-doula/faq/).

All of these activities have the potential to be mutually supportive or to generate tension if not conflict. What could be considered 'persuading' under the stressful conditions of giving birth could be interpreted very differently by all three parties, and sensitivity is required. It is critical for the midwife to meet the doula beforehand and discuss the role of each. It is also important that both doula and the woman understand that, should there be a divergence of views on treatment, the midwife's professional opinion should be considered and the clinical route forward must be the one that she is advocating.

Supervision

In the UK, supervision is a valuable resource in planning for the execution of homebirth. Supervisor support ranges from supporting midwives in planning for and, if needed, attending homebirth when all maternal and fetal progress parameters are within the sphere of normality, to assisting in organising and attending homebirths for women who are high risk and request a homebirth. A supervisor of midwives can be a point of contact for a woman who wants a homebirth in both the low-risk and high-risk setting. The aim of the supervision is always to protect the public by actively promoting the safest standard of midwifery practice regardless of the situation (Nursing and Midwifery Council, 2006).

Factors that need further consideration and careful planning that may impact on confidence in a homebirth situation are the timing of the decision made in choosing a homebirth, the basis for that decision and the possibility of opposing medical advice.

A woman can decide at any point in the antenatal period to opt for a homebirth. This decision should ideally have been made early enough in pregnancy to allow for careful planning. Also, any decision should have been made after careful consideration of reliable information given to her by her named midwife or team of midwives (Department of Health, 2007). In reality. a woman can make a decision to opt for a homebirth at any time prior to birth – with or without careful consideration. Either way, once the decision for homebirth has been made, at whatever stage, the midwife should make contact with the woman and arrange to meet her and her partner, if possible, to discuss the birth and make the appropriate plans.

One possible eventuality during this period is that the woman wants to proceed with a homebirth against medical advice. In this instance the midwife must discuss the woman's care with her first-line manager, supervisor of midwives and the consultant midwife for normality, if there is one in post. An appointment will be made with the woman to discuss her plan of care with the named midwife or midwives, consultant midwife and a supervisor of midwives. Input from the consultant obstetrician must also be sought (Nursing and Midwifery Council, 2004). During all communication processes in such circumstances it is important to avoid being perceived as bullying or coercive by women and their partners. However, women must not be 'protected' from understanding the possible implications of their decisions. Women must be informed of all associated risks and what the implications could be if these risks are not considered and subsequently managed (Nursing and Midwifery Council, 2004). If there is any risk that the woman may disengage from maternity services altogether, the possible legal repercussions for any lay caregivers' involvement, in particular should a layperson embark on delivering the woman (Nursing and Midwifery Council, 2006), should also be discussed. If, despite careful consideration, a woman remains adamant about a home delivery then plans need to be made to this effect.

All relevant health professionals, including those mentioned above and the paramedic team and general practitioner, need to be informed and their involvement and cooperation sought at all stages of the birth plan and its progress (Nursing and Midwifery Council, 2004).

The stages of a homebirth are described throughout this book and are summarised in Figure 5.3.

Care during early (latent) labour

Labour is conventionally divided into three stages, or four if we include the early or latent phase of labour. The key characteristics of the stages and associated activities during each are summarised in Figure 5.4.

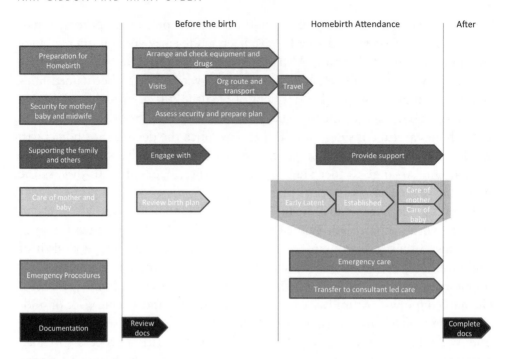

Figure 5.3 The stages of a homebirth.

Recognition of the onset of labour is not always easy. A woman who perceives herself to be in labour may not be. Sound midwifery judgement about the physiological process of early latent, first stage and second stage of labour will enable the midwife to accurately identify these stages. This section deals with the process for deciding when a midwife should attend the woman's home, the observations and actions required during early latent labour, the options for coping with pain and discomfort at this stage, and the documentation that should be maintained.

The latent phase remains poorly understood and is controversial. Labour does not neatly divide into obvious and distinct stages. It is a complex phenomenon of interdependent physical, hormonal and emotional changes, which can vary enormously between individual women (Frye, 2004). There is no real consensus about the length and specific characteristics of early latent labour. Despite these ambiguities, the National Institute for Health and Clinical Excellence (NICE) acknowledge its existence and defines early latent labour as a period of time, not necessarily continuous, during which there are painful contractions and there is some cervical change, including cervical effacement and dilatation up to 4 cm (NICE, 2007).

Careful arrangements around how and when to call the midwife when labour starts should be discussed in the antenatal period. An on-call rota for delivery should be available from around 37 weeks; this should be explained

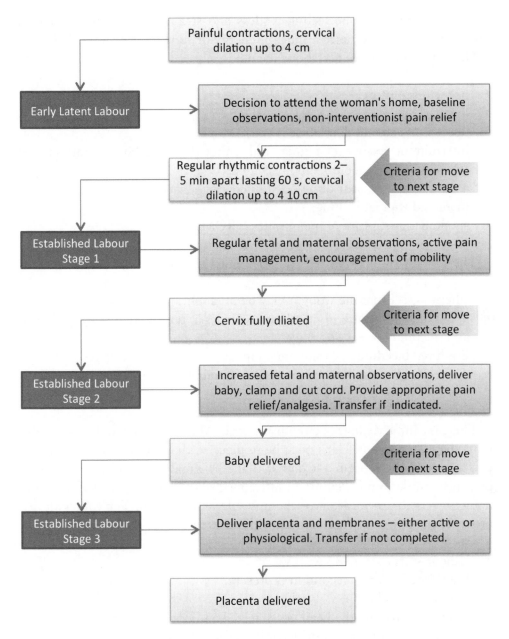

FIGURE 5.4 The key characteristics of the stages and associated activities during labour.

to the woman and her partner, who should be given a copy. Appropriate contact numbers will be given from the onset of pregnancy with explanations of whom to contact in daytime hours and whom at weekends and during the night, as these may differ.

Women often describe feeling restless and strange before labour begins. They sometimes experience a spurt of energy or start to nest (Burvill, 2002). Physical symptoms of prelabour include:

- pelvic discomfort;
- low backache;
- upset stomach and diarrhoea;
- intermittent episode of regular tightening (Braxton Hicks contractions) for days or weeks before labour begins;
- a show, which is clear or blood-stained loss – expulsion of the operculum;
- increased vaginal leaking;
- spontaneous rupture of membranes (SROM).

The woman and her partner should contact the midwifery team if:

- They suspect that the woman may be in labour.
- Spontaneous rupture of membranes occurs at term with an engaged head and the fluid is clear and pink.
- Fresh red bleeding per vaginam happens.
- There are strong painful contractions coming every three to five minutes and lasting for a minute.

There is a limited range of circumstances in which the woman should receive immediate assessment. Plans must be in place so that the woman knows who to call should these occur – whether that is the midwife, midwifery-led unit or consultant-led unit. Planning must consider the locations of the woman's home in relation to location of the midwife and hospital. The following list provides examples of when such immediate attention should be sought:

- Labour starts before 37 weeks.
- SROM occurs and meconium is present.
- SROM occurs before 37 weeks.
- SROM occurs and the head not engaged and not labouring.
- There is bleeding that is sufficient to soak a sanitary pad.
- Fetal movements are diminished.
- The woman is worried about anything that may need a clinical assessment.

When the woman makes contact with the midwife or midwifery team, it is necessary to obtain from her information that is sufficiently detailed to ascertain what is happening. After listening to the woman, the midwife will decide when it is appropriate to attend, taking into consideration maternity history, gestation, frequency and strength of contractions and how long ago they started, and whether the membranes are intact and the baby is moving. The distance to the woman's home from the midwife's place of location should also be considered.

If the midwife attends at this point, she will make an assessment of progress. Again, this will inform the midwife whether she needs to stay at the home. If contractions are mild and more than five minutes apart, membranes intact and the woman is not distressed by her contractions, a vaginal examination will not be performed and the midwife may decide to leave. If labour is not established, an explanation that strong labour is not yet started should be given. Women should be advised to try the various techniques that promote relaxation and help coping in early labour (see Chapter 7). At the onset of labour the midwife should encourage the woman to trust in her own instincts and listen to her own body (Frye, 2004). Women should be encouraged to verbalise their feelings in order to receive the support and help they need, to eat and drink as normal and not focus too much on labour (Simkin and Ancheta, 2005).

If the midwife decides to leave, having attended the home, she will advise the woman and her partner when to call again. Information will be reiterated around safety and fetal well-being, in particular around what to do if membranes rupture and the liquor is not clear, or if they are already ruptured and the fluid changes colour, or if there is heavy bleeding or diminished fetal movements. If the woman does not call within an agreed timeframe, then an arrangement should be made with the family for the midwife to return and review the situation. A midwife remaining in the home when she is not required will not help an early labouring woman or her family. A few visits may be necessary before the decision to stay is made.

The latent phase can last for a day or two (Burvill, 2002). Intervention such as artificial rupture of the membranes (ARM) to augment labour in the latent stage is not recommended (Simkin and Ancheta, 2005). In the absence of problems, no intervention is needed other than the midwife providing the woman and her partner with reassurance, support and effective information and explanations confirming the normality of slow progress. A slow latent phase can induce disappointment and leave women tired and demoralised.

Women will benefit from rest and sleep for periods. Soaking in a warm bath or the use of a hot water bottle with help alleviate discomfort. When not resting, encouraging women to engage in activities that help distract them from the discomfort of the latent phase may be useful, such as listening to music, watching a DVD or going for a walk.

Involving the father to support the woman to be active and encouraging them to massage their partner and showing them they care will help the mother to remain positive. It will also help the partner feel that he is doing something useful, and in a practical sense this helps the midwife. During the latent phase of labour, several natural and alternative methods can be used to alleviate pain and discomfort (see Chapter 7, which covers natural and alternative pain management options).

Early labour is an ideal time to revisit the birth plan while the woman is still able to focus and is not distracted by the pain of labour. The midwife should initially take baseline observations. This will include temperature, pulse, respiratory observations, abdominal palpation, listening to the fetal heart, the frequency and strength of contractions and a urine sample. Depending on the length of the latent phase it may be appropriate to repeat these observations.

In normally progressing labour, amniotomy should not be performed routinely (NICE, 2007). The decision to perform an amniotomy should be justified and made in consultation with the woman (Royal College of Midwives, 2005). Ruptured membranes can occur in early latent labour. If the woman is contracting there is no need to do anything other than note the event and relevant history and observe the colour of the liquor. Again, a vaginal examination is not necessary unless the woman requests one and is contacting strongly and regularly.

All care given and routine observations together with the outcomes and progress from observations should be documented in the woman's handheld notes. The partogram should not be started until established labour has begun. Once established labour has started then all care should be documented on the partogram and in the woman's case notes (see Appendix 5.1). All interventions, drugs given and their timings and dosages, any deviations from the normal and medical referrals should be recorded (see Chapters 2 and 3).

Care during established labour

Midwives become adept at reading women's body language and behaviour to guide them when labour is moving on from the latent or early stage to established first stage of labour. Women's partners, junior midwives and student midwives may need guidance from experienced midwives on this. As the latent phase ends and labour becomes established, the contractions become stronger and increasingly painful. The first stage of established labour is normally viewed as beginning when:

- On vaginal examination the cervix is in an anterior or mid position, soft and effaced (effacement may not be complete in multiparous women).
- The cervix undergoes rapid dilation; this begins when the cervix is 4 cm dilated.

- There are strong regular rhythmic contractions ranging 2–5 minutes apart and lasting for 60 seconds.

The first stage is complete when the cervix is fully dilated (approximately 10 cm) (McCormick, 2009). When labour is established and it is time for the midwife to remain with the woman in her home, the midwife should take care not to dominate the situation: she should, as far as possible, blend into the background (Gwillim, 2009). It is important for the woman to feel she is birthing her baby. Most women will progress well when they are in their own environment, labouring in a position they want to be in and with their family (Royal College of Midwives, 2006). A homebirth experience is a deeply emotional, personal life experience for the woman and her partner and family. To enrich this experience the woman needs to feel in control and exceptionally well supported but allowed to birth her own baby (Frye, 2004; Gwillim, 2009).

Observing and monitoring the woman

Discreet observation by the midwife, allowing the woman to behave instinctively and naturally, will contribute greatly to the labouring woman's feeling of control. During contractions the woman may become less mobile, support herself by holding on to her partner or something to support herself. Instinctive behaviour often manifests itself, with the woman standing with her legs astride and rocking her hips from side to side during a contraction. During contractions the woman may seem withdrawn, closing her eyes and breathing heavily and rhythmically; she may call out or make moaning noises during really painful contractions (Burvill, 2002). The woman's dialogue may be brief during requests for help and support, for example for water or gas. During these contractions the woman needs to be left in peace (Lemay, 2000). Equipment and aids should be arranged so that they are within easy reach but do not impinge on or occlude the birthing space.

All observations that are performed should be documented in the woman's casenotes and on the partogram (Nursing and Midwifery Council, 2004). There is a lack of evidence supporting many routine labour observations (Crowther *et al.*, 2000; NICE 2007). However, NICE (2007) recommends that the maternal pulse should be recorded hourly at the same time as the fetal heart rate. Other observations recommended are blood pressure and temperature readings; these should be recorded four-hourly. If a woman is having a water birth it is advised that the temperature should be recorded hourly (Garland, 2002; NICE 2007). The fetal heart should be auscultated every 15 minutes for one minute following a contraction (NICE, 2007). The woman should be encouraged to pass urine frequently as an empty bladder aids descent of the fetal presenting part and helps to prevent postdelivery bladder trauma.

The woman's behaviour and verbal communication as to how she feels will indicate how labour is progressing, and fetal and maternal well-being will determine the frequency with which abdominal palpations should be performed (Frye, 2004). An abdominal palpation is performed to assess the lie, position and presentation of the fetus and progress in labour. This should take place on arrival at the woman's home and then periodically, approximately four-hourly, if no deviations from the normal occurs. The lie, position and presentation of the baby should be ascertained. Confirming engagement of the presenting part and measuring its descent is key for monitoring the progress of labour. Some women find this uncomfortable, so care should be taken to be as gentle as possible (NICE, 2007).

Progress should also be monitored by observation of frequency and strength of contractions and a woman's verbal and non-verbal response to them (Stuart, 2000; Burvill, 2002). Vaginal examination is not usually warranted if contractions are more than five minutes apart and last less than 60 seconds, unless the woman requests one. NICE (2007) recommends that vaginal examination should be performed four-hourly in the first stage of labour. Cervical dilation of 0.5 cm per hour is deemed reasonable progress (Albers et al., 1996; Albers, 1999; Crowther et al., 2000; NICE, 2007).

Monitoring progress of labour in the homebirth setting is more relaxed and normally benefits from the absence of an action line on the partogram. However, if local policy dictates that an action line is to be used then a four-hour rather than a two-hour action line is advocated (Table 5.1). This appears to reduce intervention in primigravidae with no adverse neonatal or maternal outcome (Lavender et al., 2006; NICE, 2007).

Intermittent auscultation

Intermittent auscultation is recommended for all normal birth scenarios including homebirth. This includes auscultating the fetal heart at intermittent intervals, using a Pinard stethoscope or a hand-held Doppler/Sonicaid device. Midwives have traditionally timed monitoring according to the stage of labour and increased the frequency of auscultation when the woman is in established and advanced labour. There have been no randomised controlled trials to support individualised time intervals in monitoring the fetal heart in relation to the stage of labour and the degree of risk. In the absence of such trials and based on medical expert opinion alone, NICE (2007) recommends that auscultation takes place after a contraction for one minute, every 15

TABLE 5.1 Observations during labour – midwives must follow local policy, but these guidelines may be useful

Observation	During early latent labour	During first stage of established labour	During second stage of established labour
Pulse	Baseline then as required depending on the length of the latent stage	Hourly	Every five minutes
Fetal heart rate	Baseline then as required depending on the length of the latent stage	Every 15 minutes and hourly with maternal pulse	Every five minutes
Blood pressure	Baseline then as required depending on the length of the latent stage	Four-hourly	Hourly or more frequently if required depending on each woman's individual progress and well-being
Temperature	Baseline then as required depending on the length of the latent stage	Four-hourly (or hourly if water birth planned)	Hourly or more frequently if required depending on each woman's individual progress and well-being
Abdominal palpation	Baseline then as required depending on the length of the latent stage	Four-hourly if no deviations from the normal	Hourly or more frequently if required depending on each woman's individual progress and well-being
Frequency and strength of contractions and a woman's verbal and non-verbal response to them	Baseline then as required depending on the length of the latent stage	Midwife will note the strength and frequency of the contractions with the fetal heart rate	Midwife will note the strength and frequency of the contractions with the fetal heart rate

TABLE 5.1 (continued)

Observation	During early latent labour	During first stage of established labour	During second stage of established labour
Vaginal examination	Not if contractions are more than five minutes apart and lasting less than 60 seconds	Vaginal examination should be performed four-hourly in the first stage of labour. Cervical dilation of 0.5 cm per hour is deemed reasonable progress	Only if required to determine descent and/or position of the presenting part
Amniotomy	Not in normally progressing labour	Not in normally progressing labour	Not applicable in second stage of established labour
Action line on the partogram	Partogram not used until labour is established	Only if local policy mandates – then likely to be four-hourly	Not applicable in second stage of established labour

minutes in the first stage of labour and every five minutes in the second stage of labour. Local policies may advocate listening before a contraction, during a contraction and for one minute after a contraction.

Using a Pinard stethoscope or Doppler device

Using a Pinard stethoscope has many benefits. First, it is the most natural method and non-interventionist, thus promoting normality. Second, it maintains core midwifery skills as a midwife has to know precisely the position of the fetus. Third, a Pinard stethoscope will pick up only the fetal heart and not the maternal heart rate. A Pinard stethoscope can be used throughout labour, but one drawback of using one is that women may find it uncomfortable. A hand-held Doppler device can be placed lightly on the abdomen, and this also allows for the mother and birth attendants to hear the fetal heart, which is reassuring. A water-resistant Doppler device can be used in baths and birthing pools. Some women and midwives prefer the simplicity of the Pinard stethoscope. Combining the use of both devices may provide the best of all options.

Variability should be considered if there are any concerns relating to the fetal heart rate. The fetal heart rate should vary at least five beats from the baseline rate over a period of one minute. This is difficult to assess using a Pinard stethoscope, which provides audibility of the beat; in such cases the use of a hand-held Doppler device is useful as it displays the fetal heart rate and its variations. If there are any deviations from the normal, such as decelerations, bradycardia or tachycardia, then transfer to hospital for cardiotocography (CTG) should be considered. It is useful to remember that fetal heart decelerations often occur in the second stage. Therefore, if delivery is imminent, transfer to hospital will be both pointless and impractical. Many units have their own fetal monitoring guidelines, which may not always conform to NICE guidelines (Hindley *et al.*, 2005). Any deviations from the normal should be referred to medical aid (NMC, 2004) and transfer to a consultant-led unit may be advised. Any deviations from the normal will be discussed with the woman and her partner and documented in her casenotes.

Additional pain relief may be requested once labour is established and becomes advanced. Midwives will support women in using natural, alternative and complementary methods first, reserving the pharmacological choices for advancing labour when pain is at its most severe, as discussed in Chapter 7.

The transitional stage

The transitional phase of labour is the stage of labour during which the cervix increase from around 8 cm dilated until it is fully dilated or until the woman experiences expulsive contractions (McCormick, 2009). Many women find squatting and holding onto some sort of prop, such as a bed pole, helps them to cope (Figure 5.5). There is often a brief lull or reduction in the intensity of uterine activity at this time (Woods, 2006). Conversely, contractions may seem almost continuous (Charles, 2009). Some women may be restless and panic and request pain relief (Downe, 2009). Many women may have the urge to bear down at the peak of the contraction. Labour stress hormones peak at this time, resulting in a positive physiological effect that produces the surge of energy needed for expulsion of the fetus (Odent, 1999; Buckley, 2004). For women experiencing the extreme pain of transition, the ability to concentrate on anything but giving birth increases (Leap, 2000). Women may manifest behaviours that are not part of their natural demeanour, such as appearing extremely agitated, or closing their eyes and withdrawing from human communication because of the intensity of the pain (Leap, 2000; Burvill, 2002). They may shout, scream, groan or grunt whilst involuntarily pushing. Women may express a wish to transfer to hospital for an epidural or for a caesarean section, but with constant gentle support from her partner and midwife will

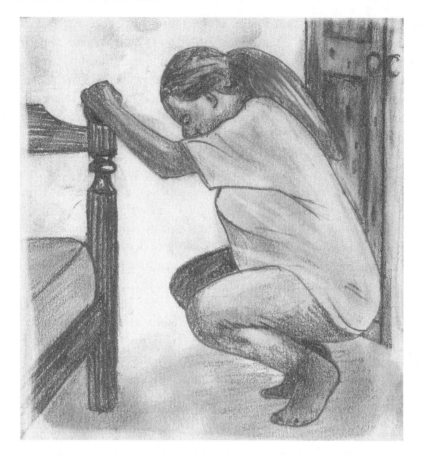

Figure 5.5 Woman squatting holding onto bed pole.

progress to fully dilation unscathed. The recognition of the transitional phase requires midwives to be tuned in to the mother's cues and use sophisticated observational skills that recognise a woman's key changes in behaviour. Mostly progress can be diagnosed without the need to perform a vaginal examination (Mander, 2002).

The second stage

The second stage of established labour is that of expulsion of the fetus, beginning when the cervix is fully dilated and complete when the baby is born (McCormick, 2009). As the birth approaches, the presenting part will become visible, advancing with contractions. The perineum will bulge and the vagina will gape. The woman's behaviour may change and she may become immensely focused or, conversely, panic and resist pushing because of fear of the associated pain. The woman may feel and display a surge of energy caused by a surge in birth hormones. These hormones include oxytocin and catecholamines, which cause what is known as the fetal ejection reflex (Odent, 2000). Reassurance and support from the midwife for the woman and her partner should remain a constant theme. Partners should be included at all stages and encouraged to support the woman throughout the duration. Second stage maternal and fetal observations need to be recorded. The mother should be allowed to moan, sob, grunt or scream as the second stage of labour progresses. Noise from all birth attendants should be minimised so that the mother can birth her baby in a peaceful environment free from distractions (Gaskin 1990; Frye, 2004).

The second stage of labour is tiring. Some women are encouraged to carry on pushing by touching their baby's head or watching the head advance in a mirror. Conversely, some women do not want to touch or watch their baby's head advancing. Midwives should decide whether to guard the perineum with one hand and flex the baby's head with the other or leave the hands off but poised ready to prevent the head emerging too rapidly. Neither action is more likely to result in perineal trauma (Caroci and Riesco, 2006; NICE, 2007). However, controlled pushing of the crowning head does appear to reduce trauma (Albers *et al.*, 2006). Promoting a calm relaxed atmosphere (Jackson, 2000), with midwives supporting the woman to take gentle shallow breaths or give small, slow pushes, can help the situation. Once the head is born, the shoulders and body sometimes deliver quickly. Most midwives await the next contraction while restitution occurs. The baby's head will turn and then the shoulders will gently emerge. This final contraction may take more than two minutes to arrive. Traction prior to this contraction should not be applied. It is the contraction that will enable rotation of the shoulders into the antero-posterior diameter, which in turn allows the shoulders to deliver.

Opinion varies whether to routinely check for cord around the neck as it is often reported as being painful (Charles, 2009). Unless the baby seems slow to deliver, untangle any cord after the birth (Association of Radical Midwives, 2000). If the cord is wrapped around the baby's neck and preventing delivery of the shoulders, then clamping and cutting of the cord will be unavoidable. Consideration must be given to the fact that that once the cord is cut the baby's oxygen supply has effectively been removed. Birth should be imminent prior to performing this procedure to prevent neonatal compromise. Delivery of the body should not be rushed. Gentle delivery of the body is as important as delivery of the head. Perineal tearing can be caused by a shoulder or a hand. The midwife will have informed and prepared the woman and her partner of the benefits of receiving the baby straight into the woman's arms for skin-to-skin contact. However, this remains the woman's choice.

The third stage

The third stage of established labour is the separation and expulsion of the placenta and membranes. It lasts from the birth of the baby until the placenta and membranes have been expelled and bleeding is controlled (McCormick, 2009). Midwives need to be competent in managing both physiological and active methods of third stage delivery. Physiological management of the third stage is appropriate for homebirth, in particular when a physiological normal labour and birth has been achieved. Again, the mode of managing the third stage of labour is entirely the choice of the woman and her partner. Active management of the third stage is appropriate for anyone at significant risk of postpartum haemorrhage as there is evidence that it can reduce blood loss and anaemia following birth (Begley *et al.*, 2010). The woman should be given information antenatally to help her make an informed choice. There are some adverse effects which need to be discussed with the woman, such as the risk of high blood pressure, nausea, vomiting and after-pains necessitating the use of pain relief after birth. More research is needed to investigate whether a uterotonic might reduce severe bleeding without reducing the baby's blood volume. Delay in clamping the cord may increase neonatal haemoglobin and haematocrit without significantly increasing symptomatic polycythaemia or jaundice (Mercer, 2001; Hutton and Hassan, 2007). This may also reduce the incidence of fetomaternal transfusion. Although delay in clamping the cord is associated with physiological management of third stage, it can form part of active management and the benefits should be discussed with women and their partners. WHO (2007) now recommends active management with delayed cord clamping.

Physiological third stage

For physiological third stage, non-intervention in the natural process of events is key. Charles (2009) advocates 'watchful waiting'. The woman should be supported to expel her placenta when she feels naturally ready to do so. Encourage skin-to-skin contact between mother and baby and early breast-feeding. The baby will probably naturally search at the breast, which encourages the natural release of oxytocin. Leave the mother and the baby in close contact and feeding for approximately 20–30 minutes. It is important not to administer an oxytocic drug or to palpate the fundus of the uterus. The cord should not be routinely clamped and cut or controlled traction applied. If the mother and baby need to be separated for neonatal resuscitation or to transfer the woman from a pool to bed then clamping and then cutting the baby's end of the cord and leaving the maternal end of the cord to bleed should be considered. The mother may experience a period-type pain together with an urge to push. Adopting an upright position to assist gravity may help the mother to birth her placenta. A quiet and relaxed environment will help increase the mother's oxytocin levels. Several attempts at maternal pushing may be needed before the placenta delivers. If the placenta fails to deliver after several attempts, then different positions should be tried, continuing with breast-feeding and encouraging the mother to pass urine. If the placenta still fails to deliver, the midwife may need the check that the placenta has fully separated or it is not sitting in the vagina. Approximately 95 per cent of women experiencing physiological third stage deliver their placenta within one hour (NICE, 2007). NICE (2007) recommends proceeding to active management after one hour. However, this recommendation is based on evidence reported by one American study undertaken two decades ago (Combs and Laros, 1991). The researchers found that the risk of postpartum haemorrhage rises after 30 minutes and peaks at 75 minutes with both active and physiological management.

There are some critical aspects of midwifery care for physiological third stage. These are summarised in Table 5.2.

TABLE 5.2 Dos and don'ts of the physiological third stage

Do	Don't
Encourage skin-to-skin contact	Administer an oxytocic drug
Encourage breast-feeding to increase oxytocin levels	Palpate the uterus
Encourage self-stimulation of nipples to help release oxytocin	Apply cord traction
Wait approximately 20–30 minutes, watching for a trickle of blood, perhaps with the presence of small clots and lengthening of the cord (signs of separation). The placenta may become visible at the vagina. Observe the woman's behaviour: she may experience a period-type pain and groan with an urge to push (it is more effective to push with a contraction, so assist the mother to adopt an upright position – either squatting, sitting or kneeling will help her birth her placenta). Ninety-five per cent of women will deliver the placenta within one hour of physiological third stage (NICE, 2007)	Routinely clamp and cut the cord. If possible wait until the cord has stopped pulsating so that the baby receives plenty of maternal blood, unless the situation is urgent

Active management of third stage

Active management will normally result in delivery of the placental and membranes within ten minutes of birth reducing initial blood loss. A prophylactic oxytocic drug is administered as the baby's shoulders are born or immediately following the birth of the baby. Syntometrine is the most common drug used, although NICE recommends oxytocin (Syntocinon 10 IU intramuscularly). This appears to reduce the incidence of retained placenta and is as effective as Syntometrine. Delayed clamping and cutting of the cord until at least an oxytocic has taken effect makes sense and confers the benefits discussed above.

The placenta will be delivered by controlled cord traction applied several minutes after the administration of the oxytocic. Many midwives await for signs of separation of the placenta first. Controlled cord traction is performed by placing one hand gently but firmly over the lower uterine area, thus guarding the uterus, and gently pulling the placenta with the other. Retained placenta is defined as a placenta undelivered after 30 minutes of active management. The risk of postpartum haemorrhage is more prevalent after this time (Royal College of Obstetricians and Gynaecologists, 2009).

Midwives need to be competent in recognising and managing any problems that may arise with the third stage of labour. Sometimes the placenta will deliver uneventfully but some of the membranes become trapped. If this happens, the woman should be encouraged to cough, which normally releases the membranes and they slide out of the vagina. If this proves unsuccessful, the placenta may be moved up and down or gently twisted to coax it out (Davis, 1997). If bleeding becomes heavy then a contraction should be stimulated (rubbed up). An oxytocic according to local policy should be administered. Syntocinon may be chosen over Syntometrine/ergometrine as ergometrine can cause the cervix to close (Crafter, 2002). However, ergometrine is faster acting. If the placenta does not deliver and all above measures have been attempted then transfer to hospital for manual removal of placenta will be necessary.

Postnatal care

Women's responses to the birth may vary enormously (Frye, 2004). If all parameters of the birth experience are normal then the mother and partner should be left to introduce themselves to their baby and discover the sex of their infant for themselves. Encouragement to continue with skin-to-skin contact and breast-feeding should be encouraged. The mother may need some support with latching, but most babies will root towards the breast and suckle when they are ready.

While the parents are getting to know their baby with some refreshments, the midwife can carry on with a range of activities that need to be completed before she leaves the home. The placenta and membranes can be checked for correct anatomy and structure, for example the presence of three cord vessels, amnion, chorion and central insertion of cord, and for completeness, that is, that no cotyledons or part of the membranes are missing.

Documentation may be completed at this time while the midwife relaxes a little with a well-earned drink. Labour and delivery documentation, including the partogram, should be completed. The birth notification and baby NHS number will normally be generated at this point. Documentation will include both written and computer-based modes. Midwives may have access to laptops to input their data or may have to return to the maternity unit to complete their documentation.

Any used equipment can be cleaned and replenished at this point. Some restocking may need to be completed back at the maternity unit. All relevant colleagues should be contacted and informed that the mother has delivered; this can include relevant handover of information in preparation for the next home visit.

Once the mother and partner have had some private time, early physiological observations should be performed. This should include ensuring a well-contracted uterus, assessment of vaginal blood loss and a gentle inspection of the genital tract to inspect for genital trauma (NICE, 2006). Contraction of the uterus and blood loss should be assessed several times in the first hour following delivery (McDonald, 2009). Routine maternal observations, temperature, pulse, respiratory rate and blood pressure should be taken. First-time passing of urine should be documented.

In summary:

- The midwife should stay in the woman's home until she is satisfied that both mother and baby are in a stable condition and that all observations are satisfactory (not less than one hour).
- The care plan and notes are left with the woman until transfer of care to health visitor.
- A written labour record and notification of birth can be placed in the woman's main notes at the hospital or forwarded on to a named person and department.
- The midwife needs to make sure that the woman and her partner are aware of whom to contact if there is a problem.
- All equipment and waste should be returned to the hospital to be disposed of correctly.
- The midwife will make arrangements for a return visit at a mutually convenient time.

- Following delivery, a midwife who has the 'Examination of the Newborn' certificate or a GP will visit to undertake the examination of the newborn, ideally within the first 24 hours, although this can occur up to 72 hours after birth.
- Subsequent postnatal visiting is arranged according to the mother and baby needs, local guidelines and the Midwives' Code of Practice, with appropriate transfer to health visitor within 28 days.
- Postnatal visits can be undertaken in the woman's own home and then at a postnatal drop-in centre if this resource is available.

Perineal care

The perineum can be examined for trauma when the woman feels ready, provided there is no excessive bleeding. Some women prefer this to take place as quickly as possible so that they can relax and enjoy their baby. There is little evidence to inform midwives around best practice for improving perineal outcomes (Steen, 2010).

There is some evidence to suggest that perineal trauma can be reduced by antenatal massage of the perineum (primigravidae only) (Labrecque et al., 2000; Beckmann and Garrett, 2006). However, this intervention must be carried out properly and be acceptable to women (Steen, 2010). Pelvic floor exercises are often recommended as a preventative treatment, but evidence remains inconclusive to confirm or refute any beneficial claims.

During childbirth, continuous support in labour (Hodnett et al., 2011), non-active pushing, a gentle unhurried birth (Jackson, 2000; Albers et al., 2006) and birth at home (Aikins Murphy and Feinland, 1998) are associated with better perineal outcomes.

Birth position may also affect perineal outcome, and the lateral position is reported to be associated with higher rates of intact perineum (Shorten et al., 2002). The upright and hands and knees positions (but not squatting) have also been reported to reduce the risk of perineal trauma (Soong and Barnes, 2005). There is insufficient evidence to support techniques to protect the perineum (McCandlish et al., 1998; Eason et al., 2002) or flexing the baby's head (Bedwell, 2006). Invasive perineal massage in labour does not reduce the risk of perineal trauma (Stamp et al., 2001). In addition, NICE (2007) has reported that hot and cold compresses do not reduce the risk of perineal trauma. However, women find hot compresses soothing and ease pain during childbirth (Dahlen et al., 2007).

Midwives need to be resourceful. In order to assess the perineum for trauma a good fixed light source is essential. The woman should lie comfortably with her bottom at the edge of a firm bed with the midwife positioned on the floor or on a low stool. If a small, moderate or large tear is evident then it is best practice to perform a digital examination of the vagina, perineum and anus (NICE, 2007). Consent must be obtained as this examination is often uncomfortable and extremely intimate. Gentleness and time should be applied to the procedure. With gloved hands, the midwife should use wet gauze to part and inspect the labia. The vagina, then the perineum, should be examined, followed by the rectum.

A third- or fourth-degree tear may be visualised by parting the perineum where it meets the anus. This will highlight whether the anal sphincter is intact, or slightly or seriously torn. Subsequent rectal examination requires insertion of a lubricated gloved finger into the anus and, by applying a gentle lifting motion, feeling the surface of the rectum and anus for tears.

Labial tears will heal well without suturing as the labia are very vascular. Suturing will be required if bleeding does not stop quickly after delivery or trauma is deep. In the case of cervical tears the woman will need to be transferred to hospital to enable the tear to be sutured by an experienced obstetrician.

Suturing perineal injury is carried out to promote healing by primary intention and good haemostasis and to minimise risk of infection (Henderson and Bick, 2005). However, whether or not first- and second-degree tears should be sutured has been the topic of much debate. NICE (2007) recommends suturing first-degree tears if the skin edges are not well apposed and suturing all second-degree tears. This guidance is based on very limited evidence from one small randomised controlled trial (Fleming *et al.*, 2003). Suture technique and suture material can significantly contribute to the severity of perineal pain and discomfort. If a skin-layer tear only is observed, then subcuticular continuous suturing is superior to interrupted sutures (Kettle and Fenner, 2007) and Vicryl Rapide is the preferred suture material (Kettle *et al.*, 2007). It is essential for midwives attending homebirths to be confident and competent in assessing and suturing perineal injury. There is some evidence that perineal repair workshops can be helpful in promoting best practice (Banks *et al.*, 2006) and improve midwives' confidence to suture (Selo-Ojeme *et al.*, 2009).

If a third- or fourth-degree tear is diagnosed, then transfer to a maternity unit will be needed. Such tears need appropriate assessment and suturing by an experienced obstetrician in theatre under regional anaesthesia. Failure to diagnose third- or fourth-degree tears may be considered substandard care, and this contributes to most litigation associated with perineal trauma (Royal College of Obstetricians and Gynaecologists, 2004). Good post-delivery repair care is vital. The woman will be catheterised and prescribed stool softeners to aid comfort and healing and antibiotics to prevent infection (Royal College of Obstetricians and Gynaecologists, 2004). The woman will need robust community midwifery care and obstetric follow-up (Royal College of Obstetricians and Gynaecologists, 2004).

Assessing perineal pain and healing after birth is an important aspect of postnatal care. Most perineal injuries heal well, but occasionally infection may occur and antibiotics may be required. Most women will experience some pain and discomfort and this must be managed effectively. A combination of systemic and local methods may be needed to achieve adequate pain relief. There is evidence that oral analgesia, bathing, diclofenac suppositories, lignocaine gel and localised cooling treatment can alleviate perineal pain (Steen, 2010). Women should be reassured that their perineum will heal and pain will decrease during the postnatal period but advised that if they have any worries or concerns they should discuss these in the first instance with their midwife or with their family doctor.

Care of the newborn

Immediately following birth

Most mothers want to hold their babies straight away following birth, and a midwife can place her baby in the mother's arms or onto her abdomen. A warm towel can be used to dry the baby and another towel placed around the baby when skin-to-skin contact is being undertaken with the mother. Breastfeeding should be encouraged as soon as possible after the birth, ideally within the first hour. The midwife should ensure that the baby has had at least one satisfactory feed before leaving the mother.

Most babies born at home are healthy and establish breathing quickly. Their condition is assessed using the Apgar score, which can help a midwife to decide if basic life support is necessary. The Apgar score was developed in 1952 by an anaesthetist named Virginia Apgar, and her surname also forms the acronym most commonly used to assess five components to evaluate a baby's overall physical condition following birth: appearance, pulse, grimace, activity and respiration (Apgar, 1953):

- appearance (skin coloration);
- pulse (heart rate);
- grimace response (reflex irritability);
- activity (muscle tone);
- respiration (breathing).

This assessment is undertaken at one minute and repeated at five minutes. Occasionally, if there are any concerns about the baby, then it is repeated at 10 minutes. The five components are given a score ranging from 0 to 2. An overall score is calculated, with a maximum score of 10. A baby who scores

3 or below is generally regarded as being in poor condition; a score of 4 to 6 represents fair condition, and a score of 7 or above good condition. However, sometimes a baby can take a few minutes to establish normal breathing and respond satisfactorily, and a score less than 7 often increases to a score of 9 (a score of 10 is rarely achieved as the extremities are usually still blue) by the five-minute assessment (Table 5.3).

Top-to-toe examination

Shortly, after birth, the midwife will undertake a 'top-to-toe' examination of the baby with the parents present. She will work methodically, usually starting at the baby's head and finishing at his or her toes, and assessing the baby's overall appearance and physical condition. The examination, in brief, comprises the following:

- head: observe shape, moulding, any caput succedaneum or haematomas;
- face/nose: appearance and symmetry, facial congestion, any nasal flaring;
- eyes: assess for any cloudiness or discharge;
- ears: look for any abnormalities or skin tags;
- mouth: insert a clean finger and examine palate and tongue; note any teeth;
- neck/chest: assess shape and appearance, nipples, breast engorgement, any trauma, respirations;
- abdomen: assess shape and appearance, any signs of hernias;
- cord stump: confirm that there are three blood vessels in the cord (two arteries, one vein);
- genitalia: appearance, passing of urine, gender, in boys assess for hypospadias, hydrocele, if testes have descended; in girls any mucous or blood-tinged discharge;

TABLE **5.3** Apgar score chart

Criterion	Score		
	0	*1*	*2*
Appearance (colour)	Blue or pale	Blue extremities, pink body	Body and extremities pink
Pulse (heart rate)	Absent	< 100 beats/min	> 100 beats/min
Grimace (reflex irritability)	None	Grimace (weak cry)	Strong cry
Activity (muscle tone)	None	Some flexion	Flexed limbs
Respiration (breathing)	Absent	Irregular gasping	Strong cry

- anus: assess for any abnormalities, passing of meconium;
- spine: examine the vertebrae, note any dimples or abnormalities such as spina bifida;
- limbs: assess appearance and symmetry, check palmar creases and number of fingers and toe; note any abnormalities such as extra digit, talipes or webbing;
- skin: observe temperature, general appearance, any birth trauma, bruising, birth marks (Mongolian blue spot), rashes;
- general appearance: assess the five components relating to the Apgar score;
- weight: weigh (electronic scales) for a baseline and detect a low birth weight or macrosomia;
- length and head circumference: measure baby length (optional) and head circumference for a baseline measurement.

Cause for concern

Any baby who gives the midwife cause for concern should be transferred immediately to hospital. If necessary, emergency neonatal resuscitation should be commenced. The Apgar score assessment should continue to be recorded every five minutes until the baby's condition is stable and document the time of the onset of regular respirations recorded.

Vitamin K

Haemorrhagic disease of the newborn (HDN) is rare but nevertheless can be serious and is associated with low levels of vitamin K. Intramuscular and oral vitamin K (2 mg in 0.2 ml) should be offered according to local policy and maternal choice; consent or refusal needs to be recorded in the notes. The midwife should discuss and give an information leaflet during the antenatal period and then again after birth. NICE (2006) recommend that parents should be firstly offered intramuscular vitamin K then an oral preparation as a second option.

First newborn examination

Usually, the 'examination of the newborn' is undertaken within 72 hours of birth by a midwife who has successfully undertaken further education and training as is qualified to do so or by a general practitioner. This examination involves a more detailed physical examination and builds upon the 'top-to-toe' initial examination. Figure 5.6 shows what is assessed and recorded.

Examination of the Newborn

Name:

Address:

Hospital number: **NHS number:**

Gestational age at birth:

Date and time of birth:

Date of examination:

Parents' consent given   Yes   No

If no reason and who has been informed
....

Head (fontanelles)..

Face (nose/ears)...

Eyes ....

Mouth ....

Neck/clavicles...

Spine...

Heart/femoral pulse ....

Lungs...

Abdomen (umbilical cord)...

Limbs (hands/feet/digits)...

Hips..

Genitalia...

Anus..

Central nervous system (tone/behaviour/movements/posture/cry)..

Figure 5.6 Examination of the newborn.

Feeding:	Breast .... Formula	
Passed urine	Yes	No
Passed meconium	Yes	No
Appearance..		
Temperature..		
Skin (colour/birth marks)..		
Need to refer	Yes	no
Referred by...		

FIGURE 5.6 (continued)

Newborn screening

With the parents' consent, the neonatal blood spot test (previously referred to as the Guthrie test) will be carried out between five and eight days following birth and the neonatal hearing test within the next few weeks. Any babies considered at risk of an infection such as tuberculosis should be referred to the appropriate health care professional for further tests and vaccination.

Recently, an e-Module for Newborn Screening has been developed to enable midwives and students to keep up to date and offer women and families informed screening choices. This web-based learning module is available at: http://cpd.screening.nhs.uk/elearning.

Conclusions

This chapter has reviewed the childbirth process to enable midwives to reflect on the physiology of labour and birth. This will help midwives to observe normal and identify abnormal labour and birth in a home setting. Preparation and knowing how to support a woman during early and established labour are important aspects of midwifery care. This chapter has focused on normal birth; abnormal birth and possible emergences will be covered in the next chapter. Midwives have 'sussing out skills' and are adept at reading a woman's body language and behaviour to help guide them as to when labour is progressing from the early (latent) stage to the established first stage of labour. Midwives are the lead professional for low-risk women and attend homebirths, but some may lack confidence and experience if most of their career has been spent in the hospital environment. It is envisaged that this chapter will help midwives reflect on their own attitudes and beliefs towards homebirth and increase their confidence to attend homebirths and give individualised care for the mother and baby.

References

Aikins Murphy, P. and Feinland, J.B. (1998) Perineal outcomes in a home birth setting. *Birth*, 25, 226–34.

Albers, L.L. (1999) The duration of labour in healthy women. *Journal of Perinatology*, 19, 114–19.

Albers, L.L., Schiff, M. and Gorwoda, J.G. (1996) The length of active labour in normal pregnancies. *Obstetrics and Gynecology*, 87, 355–9.

Albers, L.L., Sedler, K.D., Bedrick, E.J., Teaf, D. and Peralta, P. (2006) Factors related to genital tract trauma in normal spontaneous vaginal births. *Birth*, 33, 94–100.

Apgar, V. (1953) A proposal for a new method of evaluation of the newborn infant. *Current Research in Anesthesia and Analgesia*, 32, 260–7.

Association of Radical Midwives (2000) Association of Radical Midwives Nettalk: checking for cord. *Midwifery Matters*, 87, 28–30.

Banks, E, Pardanani, S, King, M, Chudnoff, S., Damus, K. and Freda, M.C. (2006) A surgical skills laboratory improves residents' knowledge and performance of episiotomy repair. *American Journal of Obstetrics and Gynecology*, 195, 1463–7.

Beckmann, M.M. and Garrett, A.J. (2006) Antenatal perineal massage for reducing perineal trauma. *Cochrane Database of Systematic Reviews,* Issue 1. Art. No. CD005123 (DOI: 10.1002/14651858.CD005123.pub2).

Bedwell, C, (2006) Are third degree tears unavoidable? The role of the midwife. *British Journal of Midwifery*, 14, 212.

Buckley, S. (2004) Undisturbed birth: nature's hormonal blueprint for safety, ease and ecstasy. *MIDIRS Midwifery Digest*, 14, 253–7.

Burvill, S, (2002) Midwifery diagnosis of labour onset. *British Journal of Midwifery*, 10, 600–5.

Cannon, W.B. (1915) *Bodily Changes in Pain, Hunger, Fear, and Rage*. New York: Appleton-Century-Crofts.

Caroci, A. and Reisco, M. (2006) A comparison of 'hands off' vs 'hands on' for decreasing perineal lacerations during birth. *Journal of Midwifery and Women's Health*, 51, 106–11.

Chamberlain, G., Wraight, A. and Crowley, P. (1994) *National Birthday Trust Report: Report of the Confidential Enquiry into Home Births*. London: Parthenon Publishing Group.

Charles, C. (2009) Labour and normal birth. In Chapman, V. and Charles, C. (eds.) *The Midwife's Labour and Birth Handbook,* 2nd edn. Oxford: Wiley-Blackwell, pp. 1–31.

Combs, C. and Laros, R., Jr. (1991) Prolonged third stage: morbidity and risk factors. *Obstetrics & Gynaecology*, 77, 863–7.

Crafter, H. (2002) Intrapartum and primary postpartum haemorrhage. In Boyle, M. (ed.) *Emergencies around Childbirth: A Handbook for Midwives*. Oxford: Radcliffe Medical Press, pp. 113–26.

Crowther, C., Enkin, M., Keirse, M. and Brown, I. (2000) Monitoring progress in labor. In Enkin, M., Keirse, M.J.N.C., Neilson, J., Crowther, C., Duley L., Hodnett, E. and Hofmeyr, J. (eds.) *A Guide to Effective Care in Pregnancy and Childbirth*, 3rd edn. Oxford: Oxford University Press, pp. 210–18.

Davis, E, (1997) *Hearts and Hands: A Midwife's Guide to Pregnancy and Birth*, 3rd edn. Berkeley, CA: Celestial Arts.

Dahlen, H.G., Ryan, M., Homer, C. and Cooke, M. (2007) An Australian prospective cohort study of risk factors for severe perianal trauma during childbirth. *Midwifery*, 23, 196–203.

Department of Health (2007) *Maternity Matters*. London: Department of Health.

Downe, S. (2009) The transition and the second stage of labour. In Fraser, D.M. and Cooper, M.A. (eds.) *Myles' Textbook for Midwives*, 15th edn. Edinburgh: Churchill Livingstone, p. 510.

Eason, E., Labrecque, M., Marcoux, S. and Monder, M. (2002) Anal incontinence after birth. *Canadian Medical Association Journal*, 166, 326–30.

Fleming, V.E.M., Hagen, S. and Niven, C. (2003) Does perineal suturing make a difference? The SUNS trial. *BJOG*, 110, 684–9.

Frye, A. (2004) Anatomy and physiology of uterine changes during late pregnancy and labor. In *Holistic Midwifery: A Comprehensive Textbook for Midwives in Homebirth Practice. Vol. II: Care of the Mother and Baby from the Onset of Labor through the First Hours after Birth*. Oregon: Labrys Press.

Garland, D. (2002) *Waterbirth: An Attitude to Care*, 2nd edn. Hale, Cheshire: Books for Midwives Press.

Gaskin, I. (1990) *Spiritual Midwifery*. Summertown, TN: The Book Publishing Co.

Gaskin, I.M. (2008) *Ina May's Guide to Childbirth*. London: Vermilion.

Gwillim, J, (2009) Home birth. In Chapman, V. and Charles, C. (eds.) *The Midwife's Labour and Birth Handbook*, 2nd edn. Oxford: Wiley-Blackwell.

Health and Safety Executive (2009) *Working Alone: Health and Safety Guidance on the Risks of Lone Working* (http://www.hse.gov.uk/pubns/indg73.pdf).

Henderson, C. and Bick D. (2005) (eds.) *Perineal Care: An International Issue*. London: MA Health Care Limited.

Hindley, C, Wren Hinsliff, S. and Thomson, A.M. (2005) Developing a tool to appraise fetal monitoring guidelines for women at low obstetric risk. *Journal of Advanced Nursing*, 52, 307–14.

Hodnett, E.D., Gates, S., Hofymer, G.J., Sakala, C. and Weston, J. (2011) Continuous support during childbirth. *Cochrane Database of Systematics Reviews*, Issue 2.

Hutton, E.K. and Hassan, E.S. (2007) Late vs early clamping of the umbilical cord in full term neonates: systematic review and meta-analysis of controlled trials. *JAMA*, 297, 1241–52.

Jackson, K.B. (2000) Postnatal perineal care and the effects on sexuality. *British Journal of Midwifery*, 8, 2739–43.

Kettle, C. and Fenner, D.E. (2007) Repair of episiotomy, first and second degree tears. In Sultan, A.H., Thakar, R. and Fenner, D.E. (eds.) *Perineal and Anal Sphincter Trauma: Diagnosis and Clinical Management*. London: Springer-Verlag, pp. 20–32.

Kettle, C., Hills, R.K., Ismail, K.M.K. (2007) Continuous versus interrupted sutures for repair of episiotomy or second degree tears. *Cochrane Database of Systematic Reviews*, Issue 4.

Kitzinger, S. (2002) Why birth without hospital? In *Birth Your Way*. London: Dorling Kindersley.

Labreque, M., Eason, E., Marcoux, S., Lemieux, F., Pinault, J., Fledman, P. and Laperriere, L. (2000) Randomised controlled trial of prevention of perineal trauma by massage during pregnancy. *American Journal of Obstetrics and Gynecology*, 10, 593–600.

Lavender, T., Alfirevic, Z. and Walkinshaw, S. (2006) Effect of different partogram action lines on birth outcomes: a randomised controlled trial. *Obstetrics and Gynaecology*, 108, 295–302.

Leap, N. (2000). Pain in labour. *MIDIRS Midwifery Digest*, 10(1), 49–53.

Lemay, G. (2000) Pushing for first time moms. *Midwifery Today*, 55, 9–12.

McCandlish, R., Bowler, U., Van Asten, H., Berridge, G., Winter, C., Sames, L., Garica, J., Renfrew, M. and Elbourne, D. (1998) The HOOP study: a randomised controlled trial of care of the perineum during second stage of normal labour. *BJOG*, 105, 1262–72.

McCormick, C. (2009) The first stage of labour: physiology and early care. In Fraser, D.M. and Cooper, M.A. (eds.) *Myles' Textbook for Midwives*, 15th edn. Edinburgh: Churchill Livingstone, pp. 459–60.

McDonald, S. (2009) Physiology and management of the third stage of labour. In Fraser, D.M. and Cooper, M.A. (eds.) *Myles' Textbook for Midwives*, 15th edn. Edinburgh: Churchill Livingstone, p. 543.

Mander, R. (2002) The transitional stage: pain and control. *Practising Midwife*, 5(1), 10–12.

Mercer, J.C. (2001) Current best evidence: a review of the literature on umbilical cord clamping. *Journal of Midwifery and Women's Health*, 46, 402–14.

NICE (2006) *Postnatal Care Postnatal Care: Routine Postnatal Care of Women and Their Babies*. Clinical Guideline 37. London: NICE.

NICE (2007) *Intrapartum Care: Care of Healthy Women and Their Babies During Childbirth*. Clinical Guideline 55. London: NICE.

Nursing and Midwifery Council (2004) *Midwives Rules and Standards*. London: Nursing and Midwifery Council.

Nursing and Midwifery Council (2006) *Standards for the Preparation and Practice of Supervisor of Midwives*. London: Nursing and Midwifery Council (http://www.nmc-org.uk; accessed 16 March 2011).

Odent, M. (1999) *The Scientification of Love*. London: Free Association Books.

Odent, M. (2000) Insights into pushing: the second stage as a disruption of the fetus ejection reflex. *Midwifery Today International Midwife*, 55, 12.

Royal College of Midwives (2005) Campaign for Normal Birth (http://www.rcmnormalbirth.org.uk; accessed 14 August 2011).

Royal College of Midwives (2006) *Positions for Labour and Birth: Evidence-Based Guidelines for Midwifery-Led Care in Labour*, 4th edn. London: Royal College of Midwives.

Royal College of Obstetricians and Gynaecologists (2004) *Methods and Materials Used in Perineal Repair*. Guideline No. 23. London: Royal College of Obstetricians and Gynaecologists.

Royal College of Obstetricians and Gynaecologists (2009) *Postpartum Haemorrhage, Prevention and Management* (Green-top 52). London: Royal College of Obstetricians and Gynaecologists.

Salt, K.N. (2003) *A Holistic Guide to Pregnancy, Childbirth and Recovery: Wisdom from a Doula*. Cambridge, MA: Perseus Publishing.

Selo-Ojeme, D., Ojutiku, D. and Ikomi, A. (2009) Impact of a structured, hands-on, surgical skills training program for midwives performing perineal repair. *International Journal of Gynecology and Obstetrics*, 106, 239–41.

Shorten, A., Donsante, J. and Shorten, B. (2002) Birth position, accoucheur, and perineal outcomes: informing women about choices for vaginal birth. *Birth*, 29, 18–27.

Simkin, P. (2008) *The Birth Partner*. Boston: Harvard Common Press.

Simkin, P. and Ancheta, R. (2005) *The Labour Progress Handbook*. Oxford: Blackwell Science.

Soong, B. and Barnes, M. (2005) Maternal position at midwife-attended birth and perineal trauma: is there an association? *Birth*, 32, 164–9.

Stamp, G., Kruzins, G. and Crowther, C. (2001) Perineal massage in labour and prevention of perineal trauma: randomised controlled trial. *BMJ*, 322, 1277–80.

Steen, M. (2010) Care and consequences of perineal trauma. *British Journal of Midwifery*, 18, 710–15.

Steen, M. (2011) *Pregnancy and Birth: Everything You Need to Know*. London: Dorling Kindersley.

Stuart, C. (2000) Invasive actions in labour. Where have all the 'old tricks' gone? *Practising Midwife*, 3(8), 30–3.

Vance, M.E. (2009) The female pelvis and the reproductive organs. In Fraser, D.M. and Cooper, M.A. (eds.) *Myles' Textbook for Midwives*, 15th edn. Edinburgh: Churchill Livingstone, p. 119.

WHO (2007) *Recommendations for the Prevention of Postpartum Haemorrhage*. Geneva: World Health Organization (http://whqlibdoc.who.int/hq/2007/WHO_MPS_07.06_eng.pdf; accessed 15 August 2011).

Woods, T. (2006) The transitional stage of labour. *MIDIRS Midwifery Digest*, 16, 225–8.

Appendix 5.1: Partograms

P490A680 (LT2002) SN

PARTOGRAM – 1ST STAGE OF LABOUR

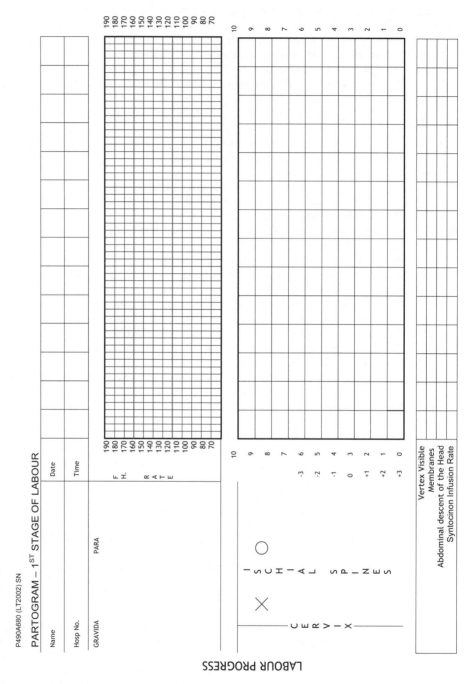

Name		Date	
Hosp No.		Time	
GRAVIDA	PARA		

F.H.

R
A
T
E

190
180
170
160
150
140
130
120
110
100
90
80
70

CERVIX
I
S
C
H
I
A
L
S
P
I
N
E
S

10
9
8
7
6
5
4
3
2
1
0

-3
-2
-1
0
+1
+2
+3

LABOUR PROGRESS

Vertex Visible
Membranes
Abdominal descent of the Head
Syntocinon Infusion Rate

P490A680 (LT2002) SN

CONTRACTIONS

| Frequency |
| Strength |
| Duration |

Position Defined

Drugs
Pharmacological
& Non-Pharmacological

TEMPERATURE

BLOOD PRESSURE AND PULSE

| 200 |
| 180 |
| 160 |
| 140 |
| 120 |
| 100 |
| 80 |
| 60 |

URINE

| Ketones |
| Protein |

MATERNAL OBSERVATIONS

Appendix 5.1 (continued)

P490A680 (LT2002) SN

PARTOGRAM – 2nd STAGE OF LABOUR

Name	Date
Hosp No.	Time
Vertex Visible	
Membranes	
Descent of the Head	
Syntocinon Infusion Rate	

Summary of Labour

Date: _____   Time: _____

Rupture of membranes _____
Onset of 1st stage of labour _____
Onset of 2nd stage of labour _____
Commenced active pushing _____
Birth of the baby _____
Completion of the 3rd stage _____

GRAVADIA   PARA

F.H.

RATE

190
180
170
160
150
140
130
120
110
100
90
80
70

Chapter 6 **Abnormal labour and emergencies**

Mary Steen and Kim Gibbon

Introduction

> There are times when we all have to face unexpected emergency and it is our reaction to such emergencies that is often more important than the sudden, and maybe totally unexpected occurrence or situation with which we are confronted.

> (Dick-Read, 1959)

Most women give birth without any complications. However, it is essential that midwives keep up to date by undergoing regular emergency skills drills and training workshops and study days so that they have the knowledge and skills to manage emergencies if an unexpected problem arises during a home-birth. This will help them to plan for an emergency and be familiar with local procedures and guidelines in the event of an emergency. However, it is difficult to access training that focuses on emergencies in the home setting. To address this issue, midwives in Powys, Wales, who practise in remote rural communities where the nearest consultant-led unit can be over an hour away have developed a training programme. This realistic training gives midwives an opportunity to practise obstetric emergencies within a home setting and encourages partnership working with local paramedics and health visitors (M. Lewis and Langley, 2007). Midwives use their own equipment which they routinely carry, and supervisors of midwives support the training (M. Lewis, 2006).

The obstetric emergencies covered in training so far have included:

- undiagnosed breech delivery on the stairs;
- cord prolapse in the upstairs lounge;
- shoulder dystocia in the bathroom;
- postpartum haemorrhage in the bedroom.

Midwives work through their actions and practise their skills, which include siting an intravenous cannula, suturing a perineum and resuscitation. This training has been positively evaluated and won a Royal College of Midwives (RCM) award for innovation.

In the UK, the Safer Births programme, developed by The King's Fund, is supporting some maternity units to lead change through a quality improvement project of their choice. Ipswich maternity services have focused specifically on homebirth and improved the management of transfers in an emergency and training for emergencies (King's Fund, 2011; Warwick, 2011). Prolonged labour and a distressed woman is one of the reasons why a woman may need to be transferred into a consultant-led unit. This chapter will review malpositions (cephalic in an abnormal position) and malpresentations (non-cephalic presentation) that may occur during labour. The aim is to help midwives to revise and reflect on the possible causes of a prolonged labour and difficult birth. We then discuss the care required by a mother or baby in an emergency situation at home, and shoulder dystocia, undiagnosed breech presentation, cord prolapse and postpartum haemorrhage are discussed here. The procedures to undertake when a woman or baby needs to be transferred into a consultant-led unit and when emergency resuscitation is necessary are also covered in this chapter.

Malpositions and malpresentations

Malpositions and malpresentations can cause a long labour and cause the birth to be more difficult. It may be necessary to discuss and consider a transfer to a consultant-led unit if the woman is becoming distressed, finding it too difficult to cope or if risks have been identified that are associated with a malposition or malpresentation. In the case of confirmed or suspected unstable lie or a face or brow presentation, urgent transfer to hospital is necessary, and it is highly likely that an emergency caesarean section will be required. However, the most common malposition is an occipitoposterior position, and in this case many women manage to successfully cope with labour and to give birth at home (Chapman, 2009).

Occipitoposterior position

A fetus is said to be in an occipitoposterior (OP) position when it lies with its back against the mother's. The occiput is in the posterior part of the mother's pelvis and the baby's head can be deflexed, which predisposes the woman to backache during labour (Coates, 2009). This malposition is more common in primigravid women, and it is estimated that approximately 10–15 per cent of all women will labour with their baby in an OP position, although the majority of these babies will spontaneously rotate before birth (Gardberg and Tuppurainen, 1994; Coates, 2009). The OP position is likely to recur in women who have previously experienced labour with the baby in this position (Gardberg et al., 2004). If the baby does not undergo internal rotation, then this is described as persistent occipitoposterior position, and it occurs in about 5 per cent of births (Pearl et al., 1993). Caput succedaneum can be present, and the sagittal suture is felt in the transverse diameter with the anterior and posterior fontanelle being palpable on vaginal examination.

Spontaneous rupture of the membranes prior to or in the latent first stage of labour is associated with an OP position because of the ill-fitting presenting part (Sutton, 2000). There is some evidence that the first stage of labour is shortened if women lie on their left side if their baby is in a left occipitoposterior

(LOP) position or on their right side if the baby is in a right occipitoposterior position as this will help rotate the baby's head to an occipitoanterior position (Wu *et al.*, 2001). Progress in labour will depend on flexion of the baby's head. If flexion occurs, the occiput will meet the resistance of the pelvic floor and rotate anteriorly to an occipitoanterior position. If the baby's head remains deflexed, the sinciput will meet the resistance of the pelvic floor and rotate forward. As the baby's head descends through the birth canal to be born, the sinciput will emerge under the symphysis pubis and the baby will be born in the persistent occipitoposterior position, commonly referred to as 'face to pubes' (Robbins, 2011).

There are some classical signs that may alert you to the fact that the woman labouring with a baby in an OP position (Association of Radical Midwives, 2000; Chadwick, 2002; Frye, 2004):

- Spontaneous rupture of membranes occurs before the onset of established labour.
- On abdominal palpation, a dip is felt around the expectant mother's umbilicus, indicating a space between her baby's limbs.
- The baby's heart rate is more audible at the other side of her womb.
- The woman complains of being very uncomfortable when lying on her back.
- The woman complains about severe backache.
- As labour advances the woman complains about severe pain during contractions.
- Contractions are irregular and there is variation in either the duration of contractions or the time between them.
- On vaginal examination you feel the anterior fontanelle in the anterior of the vagina if the baby's head is deflexed or, if there is some flexion, may feel the posterior fontanelle posteriorly.
- Some caput and moulding is present.
- At the end of the first stage of labour, the woman has the urge to push before her cervix is fully dilated.
- The cervix is oedematous because the baby's head is deflexed.
- The second stage is delayed because of the wide diameter of the presenting part.

Midwifery care

A woman in labour with her baby in the OP position will be predisposed to a long and more painful labour. Women commonly complain of severe backache and become tired and weary. They can become demoralised and disappointed when their labour is progressing slowly (Coates, 2009). The midwife will need to give continuous support and encouragement to both the woman and her partner. Here are some simple measures and helpful tips:

- Good midwifery support is needed.
- Provide a clear explanation of the situation and discuss the risk of a prolonged labour and making only slow progress while the baby is spontaneously rotating to an OA position in preparation for birth.
- Ensure that the woman remains hydrated to avoid dehydration and ketoacidosis. Offer regular sips of water or ice to suck (her partner could help with this task).
- Monitor and assess the woman's ability to cope and respect her wishes, but if she is becoming increasingly distressed and not coping well, this may indicate a need to be transferred into a consultant-led unit.
- Encourage the woman to empty her bladder frequently.
- Avoid artificial rupture of the membranes. Leaving the waters intact can assist her baby's head to rotate into an OA position and reduce risk of cord prolapse.
- Local heat (hot water bottle or warm sports pack) applied to the lower back may help ease backache.
- Back massage, focusing on the lower back and sacrum and applying firm pressure and strokes, may also help in some cases.
- In some cases, gently lifting the lower abdomens and tilting the pelvis helps women to cope with some contractions.
- Positions, encourage her to rely on her own instincts and adopt what she finds most comfortable.
- Some women find pelvic rocking, marching on the spot, or a combination of both, to be helpful in relieving pain.
- Changing position or kneeling on all fours (kneeling forward) may provide some relief from backache and help the baby's head to rotate to an OA position.
- If the woman becomes tired, it may be helpful rest, lying on whichever side she prefers and which feels comfortable.

Transfer to a consultant-led unit

The unpredictability of what may or may not happen when a women is having a homebirth has to be considered and homebirth guidelines will include guidance on when it is necessary to refer a woman and her baby to a consultant-led unit. (This is also discussed in Chapter 2.)

The possibility of, and reasons for, transfer to a consultant-led unit must be discussed with all women during pregnancy who plan to deliver at home (Department of Health, 1993, 2007). Ideally, this discussion will take place during the planned home visit consultation (at around 36 weeks' gestation).

The protective hospital environment, with its team of health professionals, theatre resource and equipment at hand, provides reassurance to the health professionals working within this setting. However, midwives working within the homebirth setting can plan well for any emergencies. This includes risk assessment and high-quality care in pregnancy to optimise fetal and maternal health and well-being. Notwithstanding the quality of care, a proportion of women who plan a homebirth will be transferred to hospital. During the antenatal period, a visit to the consultant-led unit to see a delivery room and facilities that are available can help familiarise and reassure the woman and her birth partner.

The most common reasons for transfer during labour are slow progress and the need for pain relief that is not available at home, such as epidural anaesthesia. The most serious reasons for transfer are maternal haemorrhage, concerns about fetal well-being and a baby born in an unexpectedly poor condition. Delay in these circumstances may have serious consequences. In the event of an emergency transfer, a paramedic ambulance (blue light) should take women to the consultant obstetric unit rather than the accident and emergency department. Babies need to be transferred to maternity units where there are appropriate neonatal services.

The woman and her partner can play a part during the planning stage and actual transfer when needed. Her partner could telephone for a paramedic ambulance if required. Directions to the home need to be clear and concise and the house must be accessible day and night, with good lighting. Arrangements for the care of other children will have to be planned in advance (Warwick, 2004). When a problem is identified and transfer is necessary, this should be agreed with the woman and her partner (most couples take a midwife's judgement seriously and agree with the decision). A relationship of trust needs to be fostered so that a women's desire to remain at home does not compromise a midwife's accountability to provide safe practice (Nursing and Midwifery Council, 2008). However, a woman who refuses to be transferred cannot be transferred against her wishes. This situation, if it arises, must be clearly documented, including the fact that the reason for transfer and the risks and benefits have been clearly explained and discussed.

Owing to poor collection of maternity data, comparable statistics for women being transferred in labour are unclear (Hospital Episode Statistics, 2009). However, higher transfer rates are associated with nulliparity (Fullerton et al., 2007). The discussion with women regarding their potential transfer in labour should include consideration of the distance between the birth setting and maternity unit and any other circumstances that may induce a delay in transfer. Both the RCM and the Royal College of Obstetricians and Gynaecologists (RCOG) (RCM/RCOG, 2007) believe that to achieve best practice within homebirth services it is necessary that organisational structures are shaped to fully support rapid transfer to a consultant-led unit. This includes the development of a shared philosophy and fostering a service culture in which all birth environments are equally valued. It is essential that formal local multidisciplinary arrangements are in place for emergency situations including transfer in labour and direct referral by midwives to the most senior obstetrician on the labour ward or to the paediatrician.

The midwife is responsible for transfer and must remain to care both for the woman and the baby during transfer and, where possible, provide continuing care in the transferred unit. Local guidelines need to encompass the possibility of independent practitioners providing a homebirth service. The use of flying squads is no longer supported in the event of an emergency; transfer is the only option. Full documentation of observations, reason for the transfer, actions and care taken should be recorded in the woman's case notes and should accompany the woman on transfer (Figure 6.1).

Situation, background, assessment and recommendations (SBAR) 'transfer in' form

Giving birth en route

Ask the ambulance to stop and pull over safely and continue supporting the women and her partner. If the birth is imminent then support the woman to deliver her baby. (See case study 8 in Chapter 8, 'Homebirth – born en route'.) If necessary, undertake emergency procedures and commence basic life support with paramedic assistance. If the birth is not imminent, continue travel to consultant-led unit (this may not be the one originally booked). The delivery suite should be contacted and given brief details of estimated time of arrival and any concerns. Complete an SBAR transfer in form to record observations and actions taken when caring for the woman and her baby.

Born before arrival (BBA)

A woman whose baby is born before arrival (BBA) is likely to have had a precipitate labour. The woman (if alone) or someone in attendance (partner, family member, friend, neighbour) needs to ring for a paramedic ambulance (blue light) and also phone and ask a midwife (possibly one who is in the locality) to attend as soon as possible. The midwife needs to assess the mother

TRANSFER IN Report form

This form is designed to aid good communication between healthcare professionals; please use this form and file in the woman's case notes.

Name...

Hospital number ....National Insurance Number ....

Situation

From.....................To...

Date............ Time.........Reason for transfer...

....

Background

Diagnosis and treatment to date...

....

Relevant medical/obstetric history..

Current condition..

Assessment

Airway: Obstruction   Yes..... No..... Breathing......Respirations ....../min. SpO2..........%

Circulation: heart rate (HR)........../min. BP.........Pulse........ ..ECG............................

Early Warning Score (EWS)...

Drugs/medications/IV fluids..

Temperature.....................

Partogram/Progress..

Fetal Heart Rate (FHR)..

Delivery..Estimated blood loss (EBL).................

Recommendation (plan of care) ....

....

....

....

Name.............................Designation...

FIGURE 6.1 An example of a situation, background, assessment and recommendations (SBAR) 'transfer-in' form.

and baby's condition and consider transfer in to the maternity unit if there are any concerns. In the case of a preterm birth (before 36 weeks), the mother and baby will most likely need to be transferred to a consultant-led unit (Gwillim, 2009). If the woman and baby appear well and there are no concerns, then both can remain at home and routine postdelivery care will be given. (See case study 3 in Chapter 8, 'Homebirth – born before arrival'.)

Care of a mother and baby in an emergency

This section will cover emergencies such as shoulder dystocia, undiagnosed breech, cord prolapse, postpartum haemorrhage and a mother or baby requiring resuscitation.

> in an emergency . . . a practicing midwife shall call such qualified health professional as may reasonably be expected to have the necessary skills and experience to assist her in the provision of care.
>
> (Nursing and Midwifery Council, 2004, Rule 6)

However, in the absence of medical assistance the midwife should be:

> appropriately prepared and clinically up-to-date to ensure that you can carry out effectively, emergency procedures such as resuscitation, for the woman or baby.
>
> (Nursing and Midwifery Council, 2004, Rule 6)

See Chapter 3 for more guidance.

Shoulder dystocia

The risk of true shoulder dystocia remains very low, and in the UK its incidence has been estimated at 0.6 per cent (Gupta *et al.*, 2010). However, the incidence appears to have increased in recent years, and this has been attributed to the rise in maternal obesity and associated risks, such as a large baby (4,000–4,500 g) (Baskett and Allen, 1995; Lerner, 2006).

If a shoulder dystocia occurs, the woman is at increased risk of severe vaginal and perineal trauma and postpartum haemorrhage (Rahman *et al.*, 2009). Therefore, the midwife needs to be alerted to these possibilities in the event that she may have to manage them following the birth. In addition, the baby maybe asphyxiated and need emergency resuscitation. The baby is also at risk of a fractured clavicle, Erb's palsy and cerebral palsy, and may even die (Soleymani *et al.*, 2008).

Occasionally, a midwife might find that a woman is having some difficulty delivering her baby's anterior shoulder and this may be because she is in a semirecumbent position on her bed. If this position is adopted, then there is reduced space for downwards flexion to occur when delivering the anterior shoulder. The mother's body weight can also play a part and her sacrum can be pushed upwards, thus decreasing her pelvic outlet (Lerner, 2006). In this case, simply getting the woman to change her position into the left lateral position, kneeling or on all fours will increase her pelvic outlet and make it easier for the anterior shoulder to descend through her pelvis.

However, shoulder dystocia occurs when there is disproportion between the bisacromial diameter of the baby and the anteroposterior diameter of mother's pelvic inlet. This results in the baby's anterior shoulder becoming impacted behind the mother's symphysis pubis (Lerner, 2006). Less commonly the posterior shoulder or both shoulders become impacted on the symphysis pubis or the sacral promontory. Shoulder dystocia, on the whole, is an unpredictable and unpreventable event.

Several predisposing risk factors have been reported to be associated with shoulder dystocia (RCOG, 2005):

- previous shoulder dystocia;
- large baby;
- previous large baby;
- maternal birth weight;
- maternal obesity;
- excessive weight gain in pregnancy;
- advanced maternal age;
- short stature;
- high parity;
- diabetes;
- previous gestational diabetes;
- postmaturity.

Any risk factors identified during the pregnancy will need to be considered and discussed with a woman planning a homebirth, particularly risks such as a large baby, maternal obesity and previous history of shoulder dystocia. A large baby has been reported to be the largest independent risk factor for shoulder dystocia (Athukorala *et al.*, 2006; Gupta *et al.*, 2010). However, it is important to note that the majority of large babies do not experience shoulder dystocia (RCOG, 2005) and women with no known risk factors and with babies weighing less than 4,000 g can still be at risk (Lerner 2006; Gupta *et al.*, 2010). Thus, shoulder dystocia appears to be an unpredictable and unpreventable event and can occur when not expected. A midwife attending at home must bear this in mind and keep her emergency skills up to date.

In addition, a midwife will be alerted to the risk of shoulder dystocia during labour if there are signs of a woman's labour not progressing normally.

Risk factors during labour

Risk factors for shoulder dystocia during labour include:

- abnormal first stage;
- quick labour from 0 to 7 cm then delayed dilation from 7 cm to fully dilated;
- prolonged second stage;
- protracted descent;
- failure of descent of head.

Turtle neck sign

If once a baby's head is born, it attempts to retract or recoil back into the vagina and the midwife observes the baby's chin being pressed tightly against the mother's perineum, this is referred to as 'turtle necking' or the 'turtle sign'. This prevents the baby's head from restituting in line with the shoulders (Fraser and Cooper, 2009). These observations will alert the midwife to identify a shoulder dystocia.

Emergency manoeuvres

If gentle downwards traction has failed, then emergency manoeuvres will require to release the shoulders (RCOG, 2005). The purpose of these manoeuvres is to dislodge the impacted shoulders to enable vaginal birth. A detailed and accurate record of actions taken and the type of manoeuvre(s) used, time taken, amount of force applied and outcome of each attempted manoeuvre is required (Coates, 2009). A useful mnemonic, HELPERR, is routinely used by midwives and other health professionals to assist them to undertake emergency manoeuvres to expedite the delivery of the baby. This mnemonic describes several external and internal manoeuvres that can be used when shoulder dystocia has been identified, although the order in which the manoeuvres are carried out may be different from that given in Table 6.1. For example, in a home setting, the midwife may judge it clinically appropriate to help the woman to first adopt the all-fours position, as this may be sufficient to dislodge an impacted shoulder; if this fails the McRoberts manoeuvre should be attempted (Figure

TABLE 6.1 The HELPERR mnemonic (adapted from Gobbo and Baxley, 2000; American Association of Family Physicians, 2004)

H   Call for *help*
At home, the midwife will have to act quickly and undertake emergency procedures to manage a shoulder dystocia with support from another midwife.

E   *Evaluate* for *episiotomy*
Episiotomy should be considered and may be necessary to make more room if rotation manoeuvres are required.

L   *Legs* (the McRoberts manoeuvre)
This procedure involves flexing and abducting the maternal hips, positioning the maternal thighs up onto the maternal abdomen. A partner or other family member or friend present at the homebirth can assist with this manoeuvre.

P   Suprapubic *pressure*
The hand of the second midwife or an assistant should be placed suprapubically over the fetal anterior shoulder, applying pressure in a similar way as when performing chest compressions, with a downward and lateral movement on the posterior aspect of the fetal shoulder. The first midwife should apply downward traction during this manoeuvre.

E   *Enter* manoeuvres (internal rotation)
These manoeuvres attempt to assist in the rotation of the anterior shoulder into an oblique position and underneath the maternal symphysis. These manoeuvres can be difficult to perform when the anterior shoulder is wedged beneath the symphysis. It may be necessary for the midwife to push the fetus up into the pelvis to help her undertake these manoeuvres.

R   *Remove* the posterior arm
Removing the posterior arm from the birth canal assists the fetus to go down into the hollow of the sacrum and releases the impaction. The elbow should be flexed and the forearm is delivered in a sweeping motion over the anterior chest wall. Pulling directly on the arm may fracture the humerus.

R   *Roll* the woman
The woman rolls from her existing position to the all-fours position. Usually the fetal shoulder will dislodge during this manoeuvre. Changing position and gravitational assistance may be sufficient to dislodge the impaction and may be the first choice in a home setting.

6.2). The McRoberts manoeuvre involves applying suprapubic pressure while the woman is in a semirecumbent position with her legs hyperflexed against her abdomen as far as possible to assist the delivery of the anterior shoulder, then the posterior shoulder.

Shoulder dystocia can be a traumatic experience and is associated with postnatal depression, post-traumatic stress syndrome and poor mother–baby interaction (Coates, 2009). This should be kept in mind following the birth, and extra support may be needed.

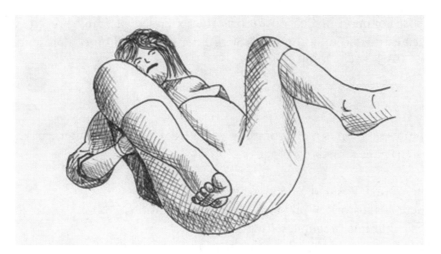

FIGURE 6.2 Woman in the McRoberts position.

Undiagnosed breech

The majority of babies present in the cephalic position at term, with only 3–4 per cent presenting in the breech position (RCOG, 2006). If a breech presentation is suspected at term, then a presentation scan can be arranged to confirm or refute this. If a breech presentation is confirmed then the mother will be offered an external cephalic version in an attempt to turn her baby and in some areas moxibustion therapy may also be available (Steen and Kingdon, 2008a). If the baby remains in the breech presentation then a hospital birth is advised and the advantages and disadvantages of vaginal versus caesarean birth are discussed. It is, therefore, unlikely that you will have to deliver a baby in a breech presentation at home. However, there is always a risk of a mother having an undiagnosed breech birth at home. (See case study 7 in Chapter 8, 'Homebirth – undiagnosed breech birth'.) This section will therefore discuss breech presentation and birth to assist midwives to care for women at home if this unexpected situation arises.

A presenting breech fetus may be in one of the following three positions (Steen and Kingdom, 2008b):

- extended or frank breech – hips flexed, with the thighs against the chest, and feet up by their ears;
- flexed or complete breech – hips flexed with thighs against the chest, but knees also flexed with the calves against the back of the thigh and feet just above the bottom;
- footling breech – as above, but hips not flexed so much, and the feet lying below the bottom.

The most common breech position is the extended or frank breech, which has been estimated to account for 60–70 per cent of all breech presentations (Banks, 1998; Frye, 2004).

Breech presentation

Breech presentation is more common when (RCOG, 2006; American College of Obstetricians and Gynecologists, 2007):

- The woman has had a previous pregnancy.
- There is a history of previous breech presentations.
- It is a multiple pregnancy (twins or more).
- There is either too much or too little amniotic fluid.
- The shape of the uterus is abnormal.
- There are abnormal growths in the uterine wall (fibroids).
- In cases of placenta praevia.
- The baby is premature.

There is evidence to suggest that a breech presentation is riskier than a cephalic presentation (Albrechtsen *et al.*, 1998). The risk of congenital abnormalities, birth asphyxia and birth injury has been reported to be increased (Cheng and Hannah, 1993). In addition, a higher rate of cord prolapse has recently been reported in non-frank breech presentations (Broche *et al.*, 2005). Thus, in particular, a footling or flexed breech presentation is regarded as unfavourable for a vaginal breech delivery (RCOG, 2006). In general, a breech presentation, irrespective of mode of delivery, is associated with an increased risk of subsequent infant physical or mental disability (Danielian *et al.*, 1996).

Delivering a baby in the breech position

Whilst attending a homebirth a midwife should always be vigilant to the possibility of malpositions and malpresentations. At a homebirth the midwife is responsible for providing emergency procedures and prompt transfer to a consultant-led unit (Department of Health, 2004).

It is essential that midwives attend regular emergency skills drills as there is evidence that doing so improves outcomes (Paxtton *et al.*, 2005).

If a breech presentation is detected during the first stage of labour, the woman and her partner should be informed and the potential risks discussed. Because of the risks associated with breech presentations and as the type of breech position is probably unknown, the woman should be advised that transfer to the consultant-led unit is necessary. While waiting for the ambulance to arrive, an i.v. cannula (16G) can be inserted and blood samples taken for 'group and save' and full blood count in preparation for the possibility that the woman will require an emergency caesarean section if there is a delay in the descent of the baby in the first stage.

If the woman is in the transitional stage or commencing second stage when an undiagnosed breech is confirmed, then it may be too late and unsafe to transfer to hospital. An emergency call should be made for back-up support and assistance. You will just have to get on and deliver the breech baby. (See case study 7 in Chapter 8, 'Homebirth – undiagnosed breech birth'.)

Remember the maxim, 'hands off the breech': if the baby is delivering spontaneously, minimal intervention is needed. However, if there is slow progress you may need to assist the delivery.

Some guidance on how to deliver a baby in the breech position

Remain calm and clearly explain to the mother what you may need to do to assist the woman to deliver her baby (Frye, 2004; Shuttler, 2009):

- Encourage the woman to adopt an upright position; sitting, standing, squatting, or crouching on all fours will all have the assistance of gravity.
- Remember to visualise the baby's position. The baby's back will be facing the mother's abdomen and during the delivery the aftercoming head will enter the pelvis in an occipitoanterior position.
- Watch and wait for the baby's buttocks to descend through the birth canal.
- If there is no progress after a few contractions, consider performing an episiotomy.
- When the baby's legs become visible, slip one hand along the anterior leg and hold the upper thigh. Next, flex the baby's thigh back towards its body and slightly outwards so that the leg bends at the knee. Deliver the leg, and then do the same for the other leg.
- Firmly hold the baby's hips with your thumbs over the sacrum and gently rotate the baby laterally (see Figure 6.3).
- Feel for the baby's arms inside the opening of the vagina and release them by a sweeping movement across the baby's face and downwards or by the Løvset manoeuvre. (Rotate the baby's body until the anterior arm and shoulder are delivered, then rotate the baby in the reverse direction to deliver the posterior shoulder and arm).
- The delivery of the aftercoming head may occur spontaneously or by the Mauriceau–Smellie–Veit manoeuvre.
- Rest the baby's body on your hand and forearm and insert your index and middle fingers into the vagina, resting upon the baby's cheeks (Figure 6.3).

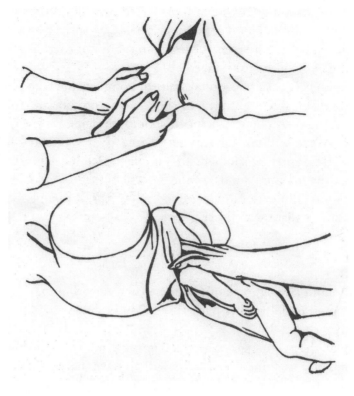

Figure 6.3 Delivering a breech baby.

- Place your index and middle fingers of your free hand on either side of the baby's neck and use gentle traction to deliver the baby's head.
- Gently elevate the baby's body towards their mother's abdomen to deliver the face, brow and crown of the head away from their mother's perineum.

Some midwives may prefer to deliver the aftercoming head using the Burns–Marshall manoeuvre. This is performed when the suboccipital region is visible and the midwife can hold the baby's ankles with one hand while maintaining gentle traction. The midwife then rotates the suboccipital region through an arc (180°) until the baby's mouth and face are visible. The perineum is guarded with the other hand to reduce the risk of the head being delivered quickly and the mother is asked to gently breathe out the head (Robbins, 2011).

Cord prolapse

A cord prolapse (Figure 6.4) can occur when there is an ill-fitting presenting part and the membranes rupture. A cord prolapse can be *occult* (alongside

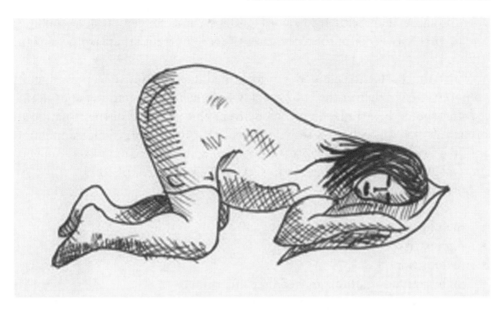

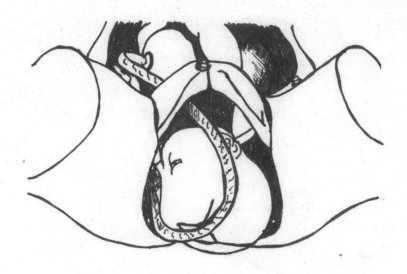

FIGURE 6.4 Cord prolapse.

the presenting part) or *frank* (where the cord escapes through the cervix and may even be visible outside the vagina) (Miskelly, 2009). The incidence of a cord prolapse in a cephalic presentation is 0.4 per cent; a slightly increased incidence of 0.5 per cent is associated with a frank breech, and incidence is further increased in the case of complete breech (4.6 per cent) and significantly increased in footling breech (15–18 per cent) (American Association of Family Physicians, 2004). Perinatal morbidity and mortality is lower with an occult cord prolapse than with frank cord prolapse, but congenital abnormalities and prematurity account for more cases of fetal mortality than asphyxia (Lin, 2006).

When this obstetric emergency is identified it is imperative to prevent cord compression and deliver the baby quickly. Urgent transfer into the consultant-led unit should be arranged and the delivery suite notified of the situation to prepare for arrival. There is some evidence that multiprofessional simulation training to manage cord prolapse is associated with reduced diagnosis–delivery interval and lower risk of caesarean section (Siassakos *et al.*, 2009).

Some points to consider:

- high head;
- high parity;
- malposition;
- malpresentation (undiagnosed breech);
- long cord.

At home the midwife should be alert to:

- cord descending through the vagina, which may be visible;
- pulsating cord on vaginal examination;
- fetal bradycardia;
- prolonged late decelerations following spontaneous rupture of membranes;
- fresh meconium liquor.

Managing cord prolapse

It is essential to call for help. Contact the emergency services and request a paramedic ambulance (the woman's partner may have to do this for you). Give clear and concise information. In the meantime, manage the cord prolapse as follows (Miskelly, 2009; Coates, 2009):

- Maintain pressure on the presenting part by keeping your fingers in the vagina and firmly pushing on the presenting part.
- With every contraction, ensure that your fingers relieve compression.
- This intervention will need to be undertaken until an emergency delivery can be carried out, and pressure will have to be maintained during the transfer to hospital and in theatre on arrival.
- This can be a difficult uncomfortable task and your fingers and hand will ache.
- Remain calm and explain why you have to do this to the woman and her partner.

- Consider the position of the expectant mother: crouching on all fours in the chest to knee position reduces the pressure caused by the presenting part.
- Another option is to help the woman to adopt the exaggerated Sims position, lying on her left side with her upper leg flexed and knees resting on the bed (Figure 6.5).
- While waiting for the ambulance to arrive, ask the woman's partner to give her fluids to drink to help fill her bladder.
- Cover her lower body to maintain her dignity.

The woman and her partner will be very anxious and afraid. Clear communication is essential when relieving cord compression and during the transfer-in and delivery. Emotional support and an opportunity for the parents to discuss their experience should be a priority following the delivery. In addition, the midwives involved in her care need an opportunity to reflect on being involved in this emergency situation and receive support from their peers and supervisor of midwives (Squire, 2011b).

Postpartum haemorrhage

In developed countries, severe bleeding following a birth at home is rare and postpartum haemorrhage (PPH) is usually managed at home or by transfer to hospital. During the antenatal period, any woman who is deemed high risk would be advised to have her baby in a consultant-led unit with a blood transfusion and blood bank service (Centre for Maternal and Child Enquiries, 2010). This preventative measure will reduce the risk of morbidity and mortality associated with PPH (RCOG, 2009).

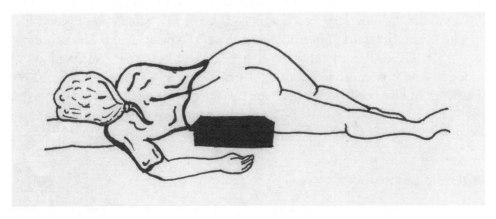

FIGURE 6.5 Woman in exaggerated Sims position. Adapted from Squire (2011, p. 108)

Women can choose whether or not to have a physiological third stage. If they opt for active management, then intramuscular (IM) Syntometrine (ergometrine 0.5 mg with 5 IU of oxytocin) is the most common oxytocic drug used at a homebirth, although the National Institute for Health and Clinical Excellence (NICE) recommends oxytocin (10 IU Syntocinon IM) to aid delivery of the placenta. It has been reported that Syntometrine is more effective in minimising the risk of PPH than oxytocin alone, but it is associated with more side-effects, such as nausea and vomiting (Enkin *et al.*, 2000). Active management of third stage is appropriate for anyone at significant risk of PPH) as there is evidence that it can reduce severe blood loss following birth and anaemia (Begley *et al.*, 2010). There may be an occasion when a woman unexpectedly has a haemorrhage following birth and will need urgent care and treatment.

> It is the woman's overall condition that should indicate to her midwife whether or not she has lost an excessive amount of blood.
>
> (Crafter, 2011, p. 149)

It has also been found that the most dangerous haemorrhage can be the slow, steady trickle of blood after the delivery of the placenta if it is not observed (Davis, 1997). Therefore, it is vital that the midwife continually assesses the woman and her vital signs and does not leave the woman's home until the blood loss has stabilised and her uterus is well contracted.

PPH is diagnosed if there is excessive bleeding following birth and is reported to be the most common type haemorrhage among women. Blood loss estimated to be > 500 ml (just over a pint of blood) in the first 24 hours is regarded as a primary PPH; abnormal bleeding that occurs from 24 hours following birth until six weeks post partum is called secondary PPH (Marchant, 2009). A minor PPH is indicated when the estimated blood loss is less than 1,000 ml and a major PPH is when estimated blood loss is more than 1,000 ml (RCOG, 2009). However, blood loss is difficult to estimate, and blood loss of more than 300 ml is often underestimated (World Health Organization, 2000). It has also been reported that health professionals' estimations of blood loss become more inaccurate the heavier the blood loss (RCOG, 2009). Thus, a midwife needs to be alert and consider other signs and symptoms. A blood loss of > 1000 ml may be accompanied by signs of shock; a woman can become hypotensive and tachycardic and may collapse.

Primary postpartum haemorrhage

The most common cause of primary PPH is uterine atony (Figure 6.6), but a retained placenta, genital tract trauma, a haematoma or a bleeding disorder

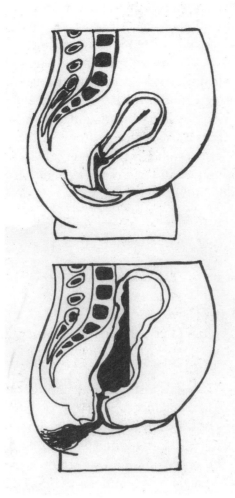

FIGURE 6.6 Uterine atony. The uterus is unable to contract, leading to accumulation of blood.

can also cause PPH. The causes of PPH are commonly referred to as the four Ts: tone, trauma, tissue and thrombin (Anderson and Etches, 2007).

- Tone: uterine atony (uterus unable to contract) can cause continuous bleeding. A retained placenta, placental tissue or infection may cause uterine atony.
- Trauma: sustained during delivery such as genital tract or a ruptured blood vessel.
- Tissue: retention of placental tissue.
- Thrombin: bleeding disorder, that is, PPH resulting from failure of blood clotting.

A midwife will need to determine the cause and act quickly. In the case of a retained placenta and abnormal bleeding, the midwife should call for a paramedic ambulance. If the placenta is delivered and the bleeding controlled while the emergency services are on their way, then that is a good outcome and the ambulance, when it arrives, can return to base. If the cause is a perineal tear, then suturing can control the bleeding but, if the cause cannot be identified and the woman is haemorrhaging, then emergency transfer to hospital is necessary. If the cause is uterine atony – which is the most common cause (RCOG, 2009) – then some early intervention steps can stop the bleeding and prevent deterioration in the woman's condition and need to transfer to hospital (McDonald, 2009).

EARLY INTERVENTION AT HOME

- In the case of a primary PPH at home, take the following steps:
- Remain calm.
- Call for help and assistance.
- Reassure the woman and her partner that appropriate action is going to be taken.
- Stop the bleeding.
- If uterine is atonic, then administer fundal massage (rub up a contraction).
- Ensure that the woman's bladder is empty.
- Administer ergometrine, ideally intravenously, otherwise intramuscularly.
- Site an i.v. cannula (16G) and administer $500\,\mu g$ of ergometrine. When administered IV, the onset of action of ergometrine is 45 seconds; IM administration can take up to 2.5 minutes to take effect. (Note that injection directly into the myometrium will have an almost immediate effect, but this rarely carried out in practice.)
- Observe the woman's vital signs.
- If the woman exhibits signs of shock, administer oxygen via a mask at 10–15 litres per minute.
- If these early interventions do not stop the bleeding then arrange for transfer to consultant-led unit.
- If bleeding is becoming potentially life-threatening, then perform bimanual compression.
- While waiting for the emergency services to arrive, take blood samples for grouping and cross-match and a full blood count and set up an IV line.
- Offer emotional support to help alleviate some of the anxiety and fear that the woman and her partner will be feeling.

How to undertake fundal massage. Feel for the fundus with your fingertips and cup the hand around the uterus and massage it firmly but gently (undertake smooth circular movement until the uterus starts to contract and feel firm). Wait and see if the uterus remains firm; if it relaxes again then repeat the technique.

How to undertake bimanual compression. Place one clench hand in the anterior fornix of the vagina and massage the fundus of the uterus with the other hand. This intervention will press the walls of the uterus together to control bleeding. This can be painful for the woman and should be undertaken only when other interventions have failed to control the bleeding and emergency assistance is on its way. Bimanual compression can also be performed externally by holding the uterus firmly with both hands and applying firm pressure (Crafter, 2011). Being alert and acting quickly will prevent deterioration in the woman's condition and manage this emergency effectively with minimum intervention.

Emergency resuscitation

All midwives have a duty to keep up to date with emergency life support skills and attend maternal and neonatal resuscitation training at least annually (Nursing and Midwifery Council, 2004). This will assist them to administer basic life support techniques and assist with advance life support techniques calmly and competently in an emergency situation in the home setting. Fortunately, in well-developed countries, where risk assessments are undertaken routinely, the incidence of cardiac arrest in expectant mothers is estimated to be 1:30,000 pregnancies (G. Lewis, 2007; Castle, 2009), and approximately 5–10 per cent of newborns need some degree of intervention at birth. Approximately 1 per cent of these newborns weighing more than 2.5 kg will need ventilation, and 20 per cent of these will need intubating (Ergenekon *et al.*, 2000). Emergency resuscitation focuses on three things: airway management, assisted ventilation/breathing and cardiac compressions.

Mother

It is highly unlikely that a midwife will need to resuscitate a low-risk woman undergoing a homebirth, but this situation could arise unexpectedly, and emergency resuscitation methods may need to be administered. Midwives must always be alert to warning signs, such as a rapid pulse, drowsiness, pallor, irregular respirations and abnormal breathing, and signs of cyanosis (Boyle and Yerby, 2011). For example, excessive blood loss from a PPH can lead to hypovolaemia if not identified and managed urgently; this will increase a woman's risk of cardiopulmonary arrest (Hayashi, 2000). An imbalance in the woman's circulatory system occurs, blood flow is diminished, the woman becomes hypoxic and carbon dioxide builds up, causing acidosis, which can lead to cardiac arrest. It is, therefore, important to maintain respirations, venous blood flow and circulation.

All midwives are expected to be able to carry out basic life support and assist with advanced life support (Boyle and Yerby, 2011). According to a Confidential Enquiry into Maternal and Child Health (CEMACH), inadequate midwife resuscitation skills were implicated in a number of deaths that were reviewed (G. Lewis, 2007). This highlights the need to acquire and maintain basic life support in all birth environments. It is important to call for help and assistance urgently. Ideally, another midwife or the woman's partner can contact the emergency services, but if you are on your own remain calm and take some deep, steady breaths, as this will help you think clearly. Before commencing basic life support procedures call for medical back-up. Look, feel and listen for chest movements. Remember the mnemonic ABC (airway, breathing, circulation) and repeat this over and over if it helps. ABC is a useful tool to help you stay focused and assist you to carry out basic life support measures (Figure 6.7).

- *Airway*. Check and clear the airway by tilting the woman's head and lifting her jaw. Make sure that nothing is obstructing her airway, for example a foreign body.
- *Breathing*. Assess rate, rhythm and depth of respirations; ventilate slowly as there is a risk of gastric distension.
- *Circulation*. If the mother is unresponsive and not breathing normally, commence cardiac compression and ventilations at a ratio of 30:2 (30 compressions to two ventilations).

It is essential that before each homebirth the midwife ensures that basic resuscitation equipment is available and is in good working order; all equipment should be serviced regularly and tested. Basic resuscitation equipment should be kept in a separate bag/box for easy access if needed in an emergency. In addition, midwives should carry a torch (a headband torch is useful), a watch with a second hand, a stethoscope and a printed emergency instructions card to help someone give clear and concise information when summoning help.

Basic resuscitation equipment for homebirths comprises:

- facemasks;
- Ambubags;

Adult Basic Life Support

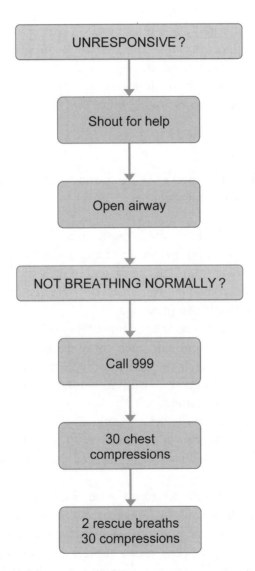

FIGURE 6.7 Algorithm for adult life support. Reproduced with permission from the Resuscitation Council UK (2010a).

- oxygen (cylinder);
- suction (portable machine) and catheters;
- cannulae and IV giving set;
- IV fluids.

In addition, the midwife needs to be aware that there is an increased risk of aspiration, and ventilating can be problematic because of the physiological changes that occur in pregnancy. Expectant mothers need an increase in oxygen levels and are at risk of vena cava occlusion if they are placed in the supine position; thus, the tilted left lateral position is preferred when undertaking emergency life support (Castle, 2009). In the home setting, use a pillow or cushion, or whatever is near at hand, to provide a firm wedge to assist you to place the woman in this position. Remember, a firm base is necessary to carry out effective cardiac compressions (Figure 6.8).

Cardiopulmonary resuscitation (CPR)

The following procedure for carrying out cardiac compressions is adapted from Resuscitation Council UK guidelines:

- Place the woman in a tilted left lateral position and kneel at her side.
- Place the heel of one hand on the centre of the woman's chest and the heel of the other hand above. Interlock the fingers to lock the hands together.
- Straighten the arms and, placing weight on both hands, press on and then release the sternum for 30 compressions.
- Perform compressions at a rate of approximately 100 per minute, depressing the sternum about 4–5 cm with each compression.
- After 30 compressions, check the airway: pinch the nose closed, take a breath, seal your lips around the woman's mouth and breathe steadily while observing her chest rising.
- Take another breath and repeat this procedure.
- Continue performing 30 compressions to two rescue breaths until help arrives. An Ambubag can be used to administer the two rescue breaths.

If available, two midwives should perform CPR and take it in turns to administer rescue breaths and chest compressions to prevent fatigue.

Once the emergency services and skilled help have arrived, paramedics will carry out advanced life support techniques. An endotracheal tube will be inserted and exerting cricoid pressure during intubation will help prevent aspiration of stomach contents blocking the woman's airway. Defibrillation to stabilise heart rate and rhythm might be necessary, and it is important to

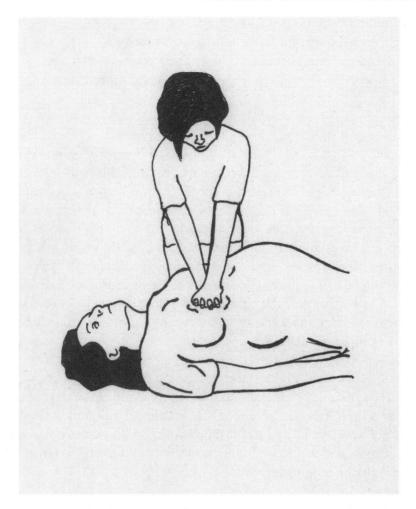

FIGURE 6.8 Woman tilted on her left side being resuscitated. Adapted from Boyle and Yerby (2011, p. 15).

ensure that no one has contact with the woman while this is being performed. It is good practice to shout out 'all clear' prior to a shock being delivered to terminate fibrillation and stabilise the heart action. CPR is then recommended under the direction of an advanced life support skilled professional, usually a paramedic in the home setting.

Baby

At a homebirth a baby may unexpectedly be born showing little signs of response or activity. Fortunately, it has been reported that only 0.2 per cent of low-risk newborns will need resuscitation (Palme-Kilander, 1992). However, the midwife needs to be aware and alert to risks that can increase the likelihood a baby needing emergency resuscitation, such as undiagnosed breech or malpresentation, cord prolapse, abnormal heart rate, placental abruption and meconium-stained liquor. Trust your instincts and sixth sense and quickly observe the baby's condition and Apgar score.

Stimulation

Quickly dry and warm the newborn as this will provide stimulation, prevent heat loss and prevent a low body temperature. This is usually all that is required in most cases. However, if a baby's temperature is not maintained within a normal range then stored glucose will be utilised to produce heat to raise the temperature; this means that the baby will need more oxygen to carry out cell metabolism (Blackburn, 2007). In addition, if a baby's body temperature decreases and he or she becomes cold, this can have an effect on the production of surfactant and increase the risk of respiratory problems (Boyle and Yerby, 2011). If the baby does not show any signs of response then emergency resuscitation should be commenced (Figure 6.9). Remember ABC: airway, breathing, circulation.

- *Airway*. Use a firm flat surface and gently lift the baby's chin to check that the airway is clear. Suction is not recommended as it can cause airway trauma and vagal-induced bradycardia (Resuscitation Council UK, 2010b). However, it may be necessary if thick meconium is obstructing the baby's airways (Vain *et al.*, 2004), and the Resuscitation Council UK also advises that in an unresponsive baby the oropharynx should be cleared of meconium.
- *Breathing*. Assess rate, rhythm and depth of respirations; if the baby is hypoxic give the initial five breaths. These initial breaths will inflate the lungs, help remove amniotic fluid and promote spontaneous breathing (Biarent *et al.*, 2005; Castle 2009). NICE (2007) recommends that initial breaths should be given using air but if the newborn does not respond, then administer oxygen. Oxygen can be given via a funnel or facemask or by cupping your hand over the baby's face (Castle, 2009). Reassess the baby after the initial breaths for any improvements in his or her condition and signs of spontaneously breathing or crying. If there is no improvement, continue administering breaths at a rate of 30 cardiac compressions to one breath (allow one second for inspiration and one second for expiration). Reassess the baby's condition every 30 seconds.
- *Circulation*. Listen to the baby's heart rate with a stethoscope. A baby who is cyanosed with a heart rate of more than 100 beats/min and who is trying to breathe will respond to stimulation and air. If the baby is cyanosed

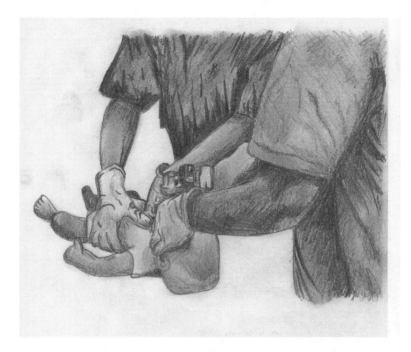

FIGURE 6.9 Newborn being resuscitated.

and flaccid with a heart rate of less than 60 beats/min, commence cardiac compressions. Use the two-finger or two-thumb method, whichever you feel most comfortable with but, if you are on your own, the two-finger method will leave you with a free hand.

An algorithm for newborn life support is given in Figure 6.10.

Some basic guidance

The following guidance is adapted from Resuscitation Council UK guidelines:

- The most common method of helping a baby who is showing signs of breathing difficulties is to 'bag and mask' once the airway is clear.
- The baby's head should be placed in a 'neutral' position to help the airway remain open.
- Observe the baby's respirations and, if these are not adequate after approximately 90 seconds, administer five initial 'rescue' breaths and observe the chest movements to ensure that the lungs are inflating with each breath.
- Ensure that the mask fits properly to maintain oxygen pressure when ventilating.
- When the baby's heart rate is > 100 beats/min, ventilation can be stopped but continue to observe vital signs continuously.

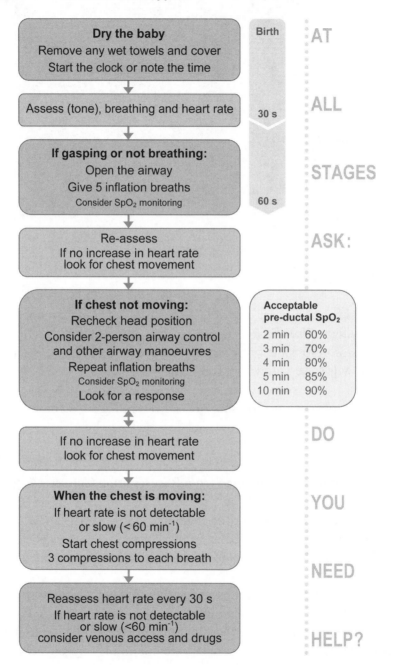

FIGURE 6.10 Algorithm for newborn life support. Reproduced with permission from the Resuscitation Council UK (2010b).

- If the baby is still experiencing difficulty in breathing and the heart rate has not improved, continue ventilation at a rate of 30 breaths per minute.
- If the heart rate is < 60 beats/min then commence cardiac compressions.

Cardiac compressions

Cardiac compressions are administered as follows:

- Auscultate the baby's heart rate by using a stethoscope placed directly over the apex of the heart or by feeling with two fingers.
- Perform cardiac compressions by holding the baby's chest with both hands and placing both thumbs over the lower third of the sternum and the hands around the baby's trunk with fingers supporting the spine.
- Alternatively, use the two-finger method in which two fingers are used instead of two thumbs. This is preferable if the midwife is alone.
- Maintain a ratio of three compressions to one breath (3:1).
- Ideally, the chest compression pressure and depth should reduce the area from the baby's chest to his or her spine by approximately one-third, at a rate of approximately 140 per minute.
- Check the baby's chest for movement. If it rises when a rescue breath is administered, this will confirm that the lungs are being inflated.
- Observe and record vital signs throughout.

Once the emergency services and skilled help have arrived advanced life support techniques can be carried out if necessary and the midwife can support the emergency team.

Conclusions

Emergencies can happen at a homebirth and transfer to a consultant-led unit may be necessary to avoid further complications. In addition, emergency skills and procedures may have to be performed by the midwife. This chapter has covered how malpositions and presentations can cause a woman to have a prolonged and sometimes difficult labour. It is vital that midwives have the knowledge and skills to care for women who labour abnormally during a homebirth and when an emergency is identified. When an emergency occurs, good transfer systems into a consultant-led unit are essential. Midwives need to remain calm, caring and confident when transferring a woman and her baby. Emergency skill drills and homebirth study days assist midwives to keep up to date, and practising emergency procedures will help them to perform these in a real-life scenario.

References

American Academy of Family Physicians (2004) *Advanced Life Support in Obstetrics (ALSO) Course Syllabus Manual*, 4th edn. Leawood, KS: American Academy of Family Physicians.

Amercian College of Obstetricians and Gynecologists (2007) If your baby is breech (http://www.acog.org/publications/patient_education/bp079.cfm?printerFriendly=yes).

Albrechtsen, S., Rasmussen, S., Dalaker, K. and Irgens, L. (1998) The occurrence of breech presentation in Norway, 1967–1994. *Acta Obstetrica et Gynaecologica Scandinavica*, 77, 410–15.

Anderson, J.M. and Etches, D. (2007) Prevention and management of postpartum hemorrhage. *American Family Physician*, 75, 875–82.

Association of Radical Midwives (2000) Association of Radical Midwives Nettalk: checking for cord. *Midwifery Matters*, 87, 28–30.

Athukorala, C, Middleton, P. and Crowther, C.A. (2006) Intrapartum interventions for preventing shoulder dystocia. *Cochrane Database of Systematic Reviews*, Issue 4, article no. CD005543 (DOI 10.1002/14651858.CD005543.pub2).

Banks, M. (1998) *Breech Birth Woman-Wise*. Hamilton, New Zealand: Birthspirit Books.

Baskett, T.F. and Allen, A.C. (1995) Perinatal implications of shoulder dystocia. *Obstetrics & Gynaecology*, 86(15), 14–17.

Begley, C.M., Gyte, G.M.L., Murphy, D.J., Devane, D., McDonald, S.J. and McGuire, W. (2010) Active versus expectant management for women in the third stage of labour. *Cochrane Database of Systematic Reviews*, Issue 7, article no. CD007412 (DOI 10.1002/14651858.CD007412.pub2; accessed 15 August 2011).

Biarent, D., Bingham, R., Richmond, S., Maconochie, I., Wyllie, J., Simpson, S., Nunez, A. and Zideman, D. (2005) European guidelines council guidelines for resuscitation. Section 6. Paediatric life support. *Resuscitation*, 67 (Suppl. 1), S97–134.

Blackburn, S. (2007) *Maternal, Fetal and Neonatal Physiology: A Clinical Perspective*, 3rd edn. London: Elsevier.

Boyle, M. and Yerby, M. (2011) Maternal and neonatal resuscitation. In Boyle, M. (ed.) *Emergencies around Childbirth*, 2nd edn. London: Radcliffe Publishing, p. 27.

Broche, D.E., Rietmuller, D., Vidal, C., Sautiere, J.L., Schaal, J.P. and Maillet, R. (2005) Obstetric and perinatal outcomes of a disreputable presentation the non-frank breech. *Journal of Gynecology, Obstetrics, Biology and Reproduction*, 34, 781–8.

Castle, N. (2009) Neonatal and maternal resuscitation. In Chapman, V. and Charles, C. (eds.) *The Midwife's Labour and Birth Handbook*. Chichester: Wiley-Blackwell, p. 246.

Centre for Maternal and Child Enquiries (2011) Saving mothers' lives: reviewing maternal deaths to make motherhood safer: 2006–2008. *BJOG*, 118 (Suppl. 1), 1–203 (DOI 10.1111/j.1471-0528.2010.02847.x).

Chadwick, J. (2002) Malpositions and presentations. In Boyle, M. (ed.) *Emergencies around Childbirth*. Abingdon: Radcliffe Medical Press, pp. 76–9.

Chapman, V. (2009) Occipito-posterior position. Slow progress and malpresentations in labour. In Chapman, V. and Charles, C. (eds.) *The Midwife's Labour and Birth Handbook*. Chichester: Wiley-Blackwell, pp. 124–6.

Cheng, M. and Hannah, M.E. (1993) Breech delivery at term: a critical review of the literature. *Obstetrics and Gynecology*, 82, 605–18.

Coates, T. (2009) Shoulder dystocia, midwifery and obstetric emergencies. In Fraser, D.M. and Cooper, M.A. (eds.) *Myles' Textbook for Midwives*, 15th edn. Edinburgh: Churchill Livingstone.

Crafter, H. (2011) Intrapartum and primary post-partum haemorrhage. In Boyle, M. (ed.) *Emergencies around Childbirth*. London: Radcliffe Publishing.

Danielian, P., Wang, J. and Hall M. (1996) Long-term outcome by method of delivery of fetuses in the breech presentation at term: population-based follow-up. *BMJ*, 312, 1451–3.

Davis, E. (1997) *Hearts and Hands*. Berkeley, CA: Celestial Arts.

Department of Health (1993) *Report of the Expert Group on the Maternity Service* (Changing Childbirth Report Part 1). London: Department of Health.

Department of Health (2004) *National Service Framework for Children, Young People and Maternity Services*. London: Department of Health.

Department of Health (2007) Maternity Matters: Choice, Access and Continuity of Care in a Safe Service. London: Department of Health (http://www.dh.gov.uk/en/Publicationsandstatistics/Publications/PublicationsPolicyAndGuidance/DH_073312; accessed 15 March 2011).

Dick-Read, G. (1959) Childbirth in emergency. In *Childbirth without Fear: The Principles and Practices of Natural Childbirth*, 4th edn. Heinemann Medical Books.

Enkin, M., Keirse, M.J.N.C., Neilson, J., Crowther, C., Duley, L., Hodnett, E. and Hofmeyr, J. (2000) *A Guide to Effective Care in Pregnancy and Labour*. Oxford: Oxford University Press.

Ergenekon, E., Koe, E., Atalay, Y. and Soysal, S. (2000) Neonatal resuscitation course experience in Turkey. *Resuscitation*, 45, 225–7.

Fraser, D.M.C. and Cooper, M.A. (2009) *Myles's Textbook for Midwives*, 15th edn. London: Churchill Livingstone.

Frye, A. (2004) Anatomy and physiology of uterine changes during late pregnancy and labor. In *Holistic Midwifery: A Comprehensive Textbook for Midwives in Homebirth Practice. Vol. II: Care of the Mother and Baby from the Onset of Labor through the First Hours after Birth*. Oregon: Labrys Press, p. 1.

Fullerton, J.T., Navarro, A.M. and Young, S.H. (2007) Outcomes of planned home birth: an integrative review. *Journal of Midwifery and Women's Health*, 52, 323–33.

Gardberg, M. and Tuppurainen, M. (1994) Persistent occiput posterior presentation: a clinical problem. *Acta Obstetrica et Gynaecologica Scandinavica*, 73, 45–7.

Gardberg, M., Stenwall, O. and Laakkonen, E. (2004) Recurrent persistent occipito-posterior position in subsequent deliveries. *BJOG*, 111, 170–1.

Gobbo, R. and Baxley, E.G. (2000) Shoulder dystocia. In *ALSO: Advanced Life Support in Obstetrics Provider Course Syllabus*. Leawood, KS: American Academy of Family Physicians.

Gupta, M., Hockley, C., Quigley, M.A., Yeh, P. and Impey, L. (2010) Antenatal and intrapartum prediction of shoulder dystocia. *European Journal of Obstetrics and Gynaecology and Reproductive Biology*, 4, 134–9.

Gwillim, J. (2009) Homebirth. In Boyle, M. (ed.) *Emergency around Childbirth: A Handbook for Midwives*, 2nd edn. London: Radcliffe Publishing, p. 91.

Hayashi, R.H. (2000) Obstetric collapse. In Keen, O.N., Baker, P.N. and Edelstone, D.I. (eds.) *Best Practice in Labour Ward Management*. Edinburgh: WB Saunders.

Hospital Episode Statistics (2009) HESonline: NHS, The Health & Social Care Information Centre (http://www.hesonline.nhs.uk; accessed 31 May 2011).

King's Fund (2011) *Safer Births: Supporting Maternity Services to Improve Safety*. London: The King's Fund (http://www.kingsfund.org.uk/current_projects/improving_safety_in_maternity_services/; accessed 31 March 2011).

Lerner, H. (2006) *Shoulder Dystocia, Facts, Evidence and Conclusions*, (http://shoulderdystociainfo.com/shoulder_dystocia.htm; accessed 7 March 2011).

Lewis, G. (ed.) (2007) The Confidential Enquiry into Maternal and Child Health (CEMACH). *Saving Mothers' Lives: Reviewing Maternal Deaths to Make Motherhood Safer – 2003–2005*. The Seventh Report on Confidential Enquiries into Maternal Deaths in the United Kingdom. London: CEMACH.

Lewis, M. (2006) One step at a time: progress in Powys. *Midwives*, 9, 101.

Lewis, M. and Langley, C. (2007) I am giving birth up the hill: will you come? *Midwives*, 10, 428–9.

Lin, M.G. (2006) Umbilical cord prolapse. *Obstetrical and Gynaecological Survey*, 61, 269–77.

McDonald, S. (2009) Physiology and management of the third stage of labour. In Fraser, D.M. and Cooper, M.A. (eds.) In *Myles' Textbook for Midwives*, 15th edn. Edinburgh: Churchill Livingstone, pp. 551–3.

Marchant, S. (2009) Physical problems and complications in the puerperium. In Chapman, V. and Charles, C. (eds.) *The Midwife's Labour and Birth Handbook*. Chichester: Wiley-Blackwell, p. 666.

Miskelly, S. (2009) Cord prolapse and cord presentation: emergencies in labour and birth. In Chapman, V. and Charles, C. (eds.) *The Midwife's Labour and Birth Handbook*. Chichester: Wiley-Blackwell, pp. 220–2.

NICE (2007) Intrapartum care: care of healthy women and their babies during childbirth. Guideline No. 55. London: NICE.

Nursing and Midwifery Council (2004) *Midwives Rules and Standards*. London: Nursing and Midwifery Council.

Nursing and Midwifery Council (2008) *Code of Professional Standards for Conduct, Performance and Ethics*. London: Nursing and Midwifery Council.

Palme-Kidander, C. (1992) Methods of resuscitation in low APGAR score newborn infants: a national survey. *Acta Paediatrica*, 81, 739–44.

Paxtton, A., Maine, D., Freedman, L., Fry, D. and Lobis, S. (2005) The evidence for emergency obstetric care. *International Journal of Gynaecology and Obstetrics*, 8, 181–93.

Pearl, M.L., Roberts, J.M., Laros, R.K. and Hurd, W.W. (1993) Vaginal delivery from the persistent occiput posterior position. Influence on maternal and neonatal morbidity. *Journal of Reproductive Medicine*, 38, 955–61.

Pritchard, J.A. and MacDonald, P.C. (1980) Dystocia caused by abnormalities in presentation, position or development of the fetus. In Williams Obstetrics. Norwalk, CT: Appleton-Century-Crofts, pp. 787–96.

Rahman, J., Bhattee, G. and Rahman, M.S. (2009) Shoulder dystocia in a 16-year experience in a teaching hospital. *Journal of Reproductive Medicine*, 54(8), 530.

RCOG (2005) *Shoulder Dystocia*. London: RCOG (http://www.rcog.org.uk; accessed 1 May 2010).

RCOG (2006) *The Management of Breech Presentation*. RCOG Green Top Guideline No. 20b. London: RCOG.

RCOG (2009) *Prevention and Management of Postpartum Haemorrhage*. London: RCOG.

RCOG/RCM (2007) Joint Statement Number 2. *Home Births*. London: RCOG/RCM.

Resuscitation Council UK (2010a) Adult Life Support (http://www.resus.org.uk/pages/als.pdf; accessed 22 August 2011).

Resuscitation Council UK (2010b) Neonatal Life Support (http://www.resus.org.uk/pages/nls.pdf; accessed 22 August 2011).

Robbins, J. (2011) Malpresentation and malpositions. In Boyle, M. (ed.) *Emergencies around Childbirth: A Handbook for Midwives*, 2nd edn. London: Radcliffe Publishing, pp. 98–9.

Shuttler, L. (2009) Breech birth. In Chapman, V. and Charles, C. (eds.) *The Midwife's Labour and Birth Handbook*. Chichester: Wiley-Blackwell, pp. 192–4.

Siassakos, D., Hasafa, Z., Sibanda, T., Fox, R., Donald, F., Winter, C. and Draycott, T. (2009) Retrospective cohort study of diagnosis–delivery interval with umbilical cord prolapse: the effect of team training. *BJOG*, 116, 1089–96.

Squire, C. (2011a) Shoulder dystocia. In Boyle, M. (ed.) *Emergencies around Childbirth: A Handbook for Midwives*, 2nd edn. London: Radcliffe Publishing, p. 133.

Squire, C. (2011b) Umbilical cord prolapse. In Boyle, M. (ed.) *Emergencies around Childbirth: A Handbook for Midwives*, 2nd edn. London: Radcliffe Publishing, p. 110.

Soleymani, M.H. Ismail, L. and Iqbal, R. (2008) Experience of shoulder dystocia in a district general hospital: what have we learnt? *Journal of Obstetrics and Gynaecology*, 28, 386–9.

Steen, M and Kingdon, C. (2008a) Breech birth: reviewing the evidence for external cephalic version. *Evidence-Based Midwifery*, 6(4), 126–9.

Steen, M. and Kingdon, C. (2008b) Vaginal or Caesarean delivery: How research has turned breech birth around. *Evidence-Based Midwifery*, 6(3), 95–9.

Sutton, J. (2000) Occipito posterior positioning and some ideas about how to change it. *Practising Midwife*, 3(6), 20–2.

Vain, N., Szyld, E., Prudent, L., Wiswell, T., Aguilar, A. and Vivas, N. (2004) Oropharyngeal and nasopharyngeal suctioning of meconium-stained neonates before delivery of their shoulders: multicentre, randomised controlled trial. *The Lancet*, 364, 597–602.

Warwick, C. (2004) Setting up a homebirth service. Presentation at Nursing and Midwifery Council Conference, 12 November.

Warwick, C. (2011) RCM's Cathy Warwick speaks about safer births. *RCM Magazine* (http://www.youtube.com/watch?v=WvyP4nYbL7c; accessed 31 March 2011).

World Health Organization (2000) *Managing Complications in Pregnancy and Childbirth: A Guide for Midwives and Doctors*. WHO/RHR/00.7. Geneva: World Health Organization.

Wu, X., Fan, L. and Wang, Q. (2001) Correction of occipito-posterior by maternal postures during the process of labour [in Chinese]. *Zhonghua Fu Chan Ke Za Zhi*, 36, 468–9 (English abstract available at http://www.ncbi.nlm.nih.gov/pubmed/11758180; accessed 9 March 2011).

Chapter 7   Homebirth pain management options

Mary Steen

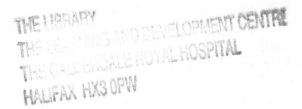

Introduction

This chapter describes and discusses the mechanism of pain and then focuses on pain associated with labour and childbirth. It then considers and discusses several pain management options available for women to use during a homebirth. First, it describes natural and alternative ways and methods, and explores how midwives can promote the use of these. Second, the options of Entonox and analgesia are discussed. Finally, the implications for midwifery practice are covered.

Mechanism of pain

Pain is initiated by stimulation of the nerve endings subserving pain (nociceptors), which form a diffuse network in the tissues of the body (Johnson, 2006). These receptors are present in abundance in the superficial skin layer and are also found in some internal tissues. Very few have been discovered in the deeper tissues and viscera; thus, pain is associated with poor location and referral to dermatomes distant from damaged viscera (Thomas, 1997; Raouf *et al.*, 2010). Activation of these nociceptors induces nerve impulses, which travel along the peripheral nerves and enter the spinal cord via the dorsal horn. It has been postulated that site is the location of the 'gate' that is central the 'gate control theory' of pain (Melzack and Wall, 1965; Rice, 1992). The 'gate' must be opened for information to be passed to the brain and for pain perception to occur.

The activity is initiated when nerve impulses conveying painful information arrive from the periphery via the ascending pathway of the spinal cord. The gating mechanism consists of two types of neurones: cells in the substantia gelatinosa (SG cells) and transmission cells (T cells). Transmission of information concerning pain is achieved by activation of the T cell, whereas the SG cell inhibits activity (Frye, 2004).

Some nerve impulses ascend to the brain by what is known as the anterolateral sensory pathway, which involves the spinothalamic and spinoreticular tracts. The spinothalamic tract is known to ascend to the thalamus of the brain and then to the somatosensory cortex of the cerebrum, where the sensory aspects of pain are processed. There is evidence that the spinoreticular tract makes extensive links with several parts of the brain such as the hypothalamus, which is responsible for the autonomic responses to pain, the limbic system, which is thought to initiate emotional responses to pain, and the frontal lobe of the cerebrum, which is thought to be responsible for the cognitive responses to pain (O'Hara, 1996; Johnson, 2006).

It has been suggested that the gating mechanism can be affected by the amount of activity in the large alpha/beta fibres that are responsible for transmitting non-noxious stimuli (Melzack and Wall, 1996; Johnson, 2006). The alpha/beta neurones release inhibitory neurotransmitters at synapses within the central nervous system whereas alpha/delta and C fibres release an excitatory neurotransmitter. According to the gate control theory, if the dominant input to the 'gate' comes from the large alpha/beta fibres, the gate will close and inhibit the transmission of impulses to the brain. In contrast, if there is an established input to the 'gate' by the small alpha/delta fibres and C fibres, the gate will open and will facilitate the transmission of pain (Melzack and Wall, 1996; Johnson, 2006). It is also well recognised that the 'gate' can be affected by impulses descending from the brain and by cognitive processes, in other words the state of the mind. If a person therefore is relaxed and anxiety is reduced, descending impulses from the brain activate the SG cells and inhibit T-cell activity. In contrast, when a person is very anxious, impulses travel from the limbic system of the brain and activate the T cells, which will increase the perception of pain (Royle and Walsh, 1993; Melzack and Wall, 1996).

Evidence to support this theory has been provided by other pain researchers, and a number of popular pain relief methods – for example, hot and cold therapy, massage, acupuncture and transcutaneous electrical nerve stimulation (TENS) – are based on this theory (Royle and Walsh, 1993; Johnson, 2006). This pain theory has gained general acceptance by health professionals. The gate control theory of pain has provided a conceptual framework for the integration of the sensory, emotional and behavioural dimensions of pain (Sofaer, 1992).

The gate control theory considers the multidimensional complexities of the experience of pain:

- It accounts for pain mechanisms.
- It takes into account the physiological and psychological dimensions of pain.
- It proposes that the complex, subjective experience of pain results from a pattern of neural activity within the brain.
- It describes how pain is initiated by nerve impulses, which convey pain information from the periphery to the brain via the ascending pathways of the spinal cord.
- It describes how a neural mechanism in the dorsal horn of the spinal cord acts as a gating mechanism through which peripheral information passes.
- It explains how information from the brain descends via the gating mechanism.

- It accounts for the fact that the activity of the gating mechanism can be affected by cognitive processes such as past experiences, attention, emotions and impulses.

Natural opiates

There is research evidence to suggest that the body produces 'natural opiates'. Enkephalins and endorphins are thought to modify pain transmission rather than alter pain perception or tolerance (Hughes *et al.*, 1975; Goldstein, 1978; Friederickson and Geary, 1982). Endorphins are present in the anterior pituitary gland and enkephalins are present in the posterior pituitary gland and also distributed throughout the thalamus, the hypothalamus, the limbic system and areas of the spinal cord. They suppress pain by blocking and inhibiting the action of prostaglandin and substance P (neurotransmitters). Enkephalins appear most active when pain is present. Levels rise during exercise, in labour and when morphine is taken.

Pain associated with labour and childbirth

Pain associated with labour and childbirth is not fully understood as yet but is unique to the birthing process, and pain sensation is different in the different stages of labour. Labour pain alerts the woman to find a safe place to give birth. Labour pain varies enormously between individual women. Some women have relatively painless labours and some women describe the pain as moderate, whereas others will describe the pain as severe. Fear and anxiety will increase tension, leading to the release of adrenaline and an increase in pain (Gaskin, 2008, p. 149).

The intensity and response to labour pain can be affected by:

- culture;
- previous experience;
- emotional state and anticipation;
- fear, anxiety, stress, fear of the unknown.

First stage of labour

Labour pain is felt over dermatomes supplied by the spinal cord. In early labour, pain sensations are transferred from the uterus via sympathetic nervous system, through the eleventh and twelfth thoracic dermatomes. As labour progresses, pain intensity increases and the tenth thoracic and first lumbar dermatomes become involved (Figure 7.1). Cervical dilation is responsible for most of the pain felt during the first stage of labour (Frye, 2004).

Pain progresses from aching to cramping to a sharp and intense sensation during contractions that usually subsides as the contraction fades.

(Frye, 2004, p. 256)

These pain sensations help guide the expectant mother to change her posture and position during established labour to assist her baby to reposition, rotate and descend, which relieves some of the pain (Sutton, 2000).

Second and third stages of labour

Labour pain during the second and third stages of labour is different (Figure 7.2). A woman's cervix is fully dilated and neural stimulation decreases. However, contractions of the uterus are maintained and the fetus descends through the pelvis. Pressure on nerve fibres in the pelvic floor and perineal region increases pain in these areas. Pain during childbirth is also caused by other factors such as stretching of the pelvic peritoneum and uterus segments, stretching of the bladder, urethra and rectum, and pressure on the lumbosacral

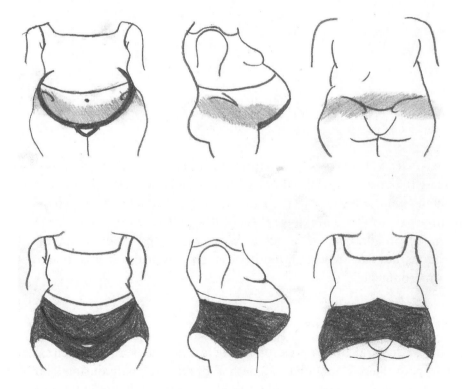

FIGURE 7.1 Pain intensity and distribution in relation to dermatomes in the first stage of labour. Top: Early first stage, pain intensity moderate. Bottom: Late first stage, pain intensity severe. Adapted from Frye (2004, p. 256).

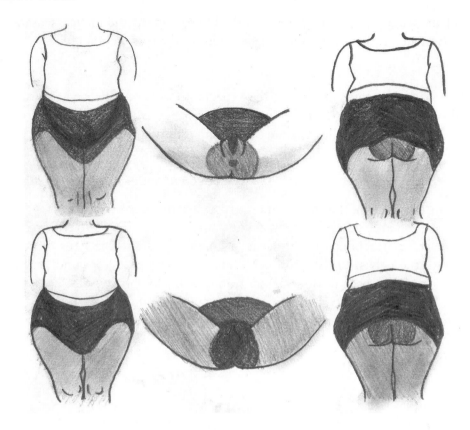

FIGURE 7.2 Pain intensity and distribution in relation to dermatomes in the second stage of labour. Top: Early second stage. Bottom: Delivery. Adapted from Frye (2004, p. 256).

nerve plexus. For this reason, a baby in the occipitoposterior (OP) position can increase the intensity of labour pain. Many women will experience aching and cramping pain sensations in their thighs during late labour and when feeling the urge to bear down and push (Frye, 2004). This is associated with pressure on the lumbosacral plexus, which involves the L2 and L3 dermatomes. These sensations alert the expectant mother that birth is near and it is time to find a safe environment.

Pain management options

Owing to cultural differences, psychological attitudes and women's perception of pain, there is no universal method of relieving pain during labour and birth. Therefore, to meet individual needs, a combination of methods may be needed to manage the pain during labour and birth at home.

Natural induced pain management

During labour, enkephalins and endorphins (substances produced naturally to help the body cope with pain) are released to provide the woman with some naturally induced pain relief. In the home setting women are in their own familiar surroundings and therefore tend to remain calm and release enkephalins and endorphins. It is important that midwives work in partnership with the woman and her partner to promote the release of enkephalins and endorphins to produce naturally induced pain relief.

> . . . one can have pain coexisting with satisfaction, enjoyment, and empowerment.
>
> (Simkin and Bolding, 2004)

A 'working with pain' approach will be beneficial to the woman and her partner (Walsh, 2006). Walsh (2007) demonstrates some key differentials between an intuitive 'working with pain' approach and a 'pain relief' approach (Table 7.1).

Companionship and support

There is historical evidence of women having the continuous support of other women in their local community during labour and birth (Brooke, 1997). Negative psychological influences such as being left alone, unkind or insensitive attitudes of health professionals and lack of knowledge in birth partners can contribute to a woman feeling unsupported (Simkin and Klaus, 2004). This will increase the likelihood of pain and distress during labour. Support and companionship during labour are vital components to promote a positive birth experience.

Today, there is substantial research evidence to demonstrate the benefits of companionship and support during birth (Hodnett *et al.*, 2011). Women who have a close support person tend to have a more positive birth experience. According to Wockel and colleagues (2007), a well-prepared father has a positive effect on his partner, which can promote a positive birth experience and reduce the fear of seeing his partner in pain. Birth support from the woman's partner, if it is practical rather than just emotional, is correlated with shorter labour and less pain (Tarkka *et al.*, 2000; M.Y. Chang *et al.*, 2002; Latifses *et al.*, 2005).

According to Downe (2004, p. 50) 'how much a man trusts other carers and how much he trusts the woman's body to be able to give birth will have an influence on his understanding and fear within the situation'. It is, therefore,

TABLE 7.1 Pain relief versus working with pain approaches

Pain relief approach	Working with pain approach
Language suggestive of pain as a problem	Language suggestive of pain as normative
Paternalistic, 'we can protect you from unnecessary stress'	Egalitarian empowerment, 'we are alongside you'
Techno/rationalism age, pain is preventable/treatable	Labour pain timeless component of 'rites of passage' transitions
Neutral impact of environment	Seminal impact of environment
Clinical expertise of professional carers	Supportive role of birth companions
Special session/focus in antenatal education	Woven throughout labour preparation sessions
'Menu approach' to options for coping with pain	Supportive strategies for journey of labour
Pain as a 'management issue' for assembly-line birth	Pain as one dimension of labour care in one-to-one, small-scale birth settings
Contributes to rising trend in epidural rates	Contributes to trend to less pharmacological analgesia
Risks of pharmacological agents outweighed by benefits	'Cascade of intervention' dynamic
First birth special case for 'menu approach'	First birth ideal opportunity for 'working with pain'
Informed choice means all options must be presented	Informed choice within context of birthing plan and philosophy

important that the woman's partner is well prepared to support her in her choice and birth at home.

Alternative and complementary therapies

Complementary therapies

Over the last decade the level of public and professional interest in complementary therapies during pregnancy, childbirth and following birth has increased (Ernst *et al.*, 2005; Tiran, 2006; Royal College of Midwives, 2007; Steen, 2007). A survey of the use of complementary therapies in 221 UK maternity units found that 34 per cent of units were providing complementary therapy services and the most frequently available therapies were massage, aromatherapy, acupuncture and reflexology (Mitchell *et al.*, 2006). In addition, it has been reported that there are several midwife–complementary therapists who use other therapies such as yoga, reiki, shiatsu and homeopathy when supporting and caring for women during birth (Mitchell and Williams, 2007).

Complementary therapies are based upon a holistic approach which notes the response of a person on a mental, emotional and physical level and gives treatment relating to the overall needs of a person. Some of these therapies can be self-administered whereas others are practitioner administered. Thus, knowledge and an appreciation of the benefits of these therapies to improve the birth experience and reduce pain perception are an essential aspect of midwifery care.

Many women are becoming more aware of the availability of complementary and alternative therapies and are also choosing to use these during their childbirth experience at home. Women can use various natural and alternative ways during their labour to help them cope with pain, and the main benefit of these is that the focus is on the woman rather than her symptoms. This helps her to prepare for labour emotionally, spiritually and physically.

The Royal College of Midwives (RCM) recognises that many women may find the use of complementary and alternative therapies during childbirth helpful (Royal College of Midwives, 2007), and this recognition fits in with the RCM's philosophy and ongoing Campaign for Normal Birth (Royal College of Midwives, 2005). In the UK, the Nursing, Midwifery Council (NMC) (NMC, 2004, 2006a,b) provides principles to guide midwives on their role, responsibilities and how to safely incorporate alternative and complementary therapies into clinical practice. Therefore, there is national and professional acknowledgement that there is a need to embrace holistic approaches as these can support normal birth practices and promote a woman-centred and holistic approach to care. Alternative and complementary therapies support individualised sensitive care that encompass a woman's physical, emotional, psychological and spiritual needs during birth. This approach fits well within a social midwifery model of care that places emphasis on holism (Tiran and Mack, 2000). In addition, the *National Service Framework for Children, Young People and Maternity Services* (Department of Health, 2004) recommended that all staff have up-to-date knowledge and skills to support women who choose to labour without pharmacological intervention.

This chapter, therefore, will cover some of the natural and alternative options available for women to use in their own home:

- being active;
- breathing exercises;
- relaxation techniques;
- self-hypnosis;
- massage;
- acupressure;
- shiatsu;

- reflexology;
- acupuncture;
- aromatherapy;
- homeopathic remedies;
- water;
- TENS;
- analgesia.

Being active

Historical perspective

Historical evidence demonstrates that women have been active during birth for centuries and have adopted squatting, kneeling or sitting positions (Brooke, 1997). A birthing stool was first mentioned in Babylonian times and became popular in many European countries in the Middle Ages (Donnison, 1998).

During the seventeenth century it became fashionable in many European countries for women to labour horizontally, and this coincided with a trend towards medical supervision in childbirth. Physicians needed to have easy access to the vagina for the purpose of examination, and in the nineteenth and twentieth centuries pain relief methods contributed to reduced mobility and drowsiness of women in labour. This led to an expectation and acceptance that during childbirth women should lie passively in bed (Royal College of Midwives, 2008). Even though there is good evidence to demonstrate that being active during labour is beneficial to women, many women still labour passively in a hospital bed. However, in her own home a woman is more likely to remain active and deliver her baby in a position of her choosing. Her home environment is familiar to her and this will promote a feeling of safety and freedom of movement. Good support from a midwife and the woman's partner or alternative birth partner is also vitally important. The option and benefits of having a homebirth should be routinely discussed with the woman during the booking-in appointment. If she chooses this option, then good antenatal preparation will support her in her decision and give her confidence to achieve a positive birth experience.

Antenatal preparation

A Cochrane systematic review entitled 'Aerobic exercise for women during pregnancy' concluded that regular exercise during pregnancy appears to improve or maintain physical fitness and body image (Kramer and McDonald, 2006). Exercise can improve self-esteem and self-image, prepare the body for the strenuous activity of labour and speed postpartum recovery (Zeanah and Schlosser, 1993; Horns *et al.*, 1996).

A review concluded that women who exercise regularly are more likely to have shorter labours with less intervention and recover more quickly after the birth (Clapp, 2001). There is also some evidence that women can exercise safely during pregnancy and this may reduce their risk of caesarean section (Butler *et al.*, 2004). Low-impact exercises, Pilates-based exercises and relaxation techniques are considered to be safe (Windsor and Laska, 2002; Brayshaw, 2003). It appears that some exercises can enhance the second stage of labour, and it has been suggested that these should be practised during pregnancy (Tupler, 2000).

During pregnancy, opportunities to discuss and demonstrate how to remain active and adopt different positions in labour will help the woman and her partner to prepare to remain active during labour. Most women are able to stay active for most of their labour and should be encouraged to do so. Midwives need to promote self-belief so that women become confident in their ability to be active during labour given that lying on a bed continuously is not good for them as this will slow down their labour. Explaining that in the upright position the baby's head exerts pressure on the cervix and pelvic floor, stimulating the release of oxytocin and promoting good contractions, so that labour progresses at nature intended, will encourage women to remain active (Russell, 2008).

Being active during labour is much easier to achieve in the woman's own home. Walking around in familiar surroundings and changing position can help the woman cope with labour pain. Using props such as a chair, bean bag or birth ball can help a woman to remain active during labour, and women should be advised of the benefits of these.

Maternal health and well-being project

The author of this chapter and editor of the book (Mary Steen) developed and successfully implemented a holistic health and well-being programme to promote normal birth practices and healthier lifestyles (Steen, 2007). The aim of the programme was to promote health and fitness during pregnancy and to help women prepare for birth and then maintain health and fitness after childbirth (Figure 7.3). Evaluation of the programme revealed that positive findings included an increase in the number women planning to be active during their labours and increased awareness of the option of a homebirth. Overall, women reported they liked exercising and gained confidence for an active birth (see www.bbc.co.uk/leeds/features/living/fitness/pregnancy_pilates.shtml; Steen, 2007, p. 119):

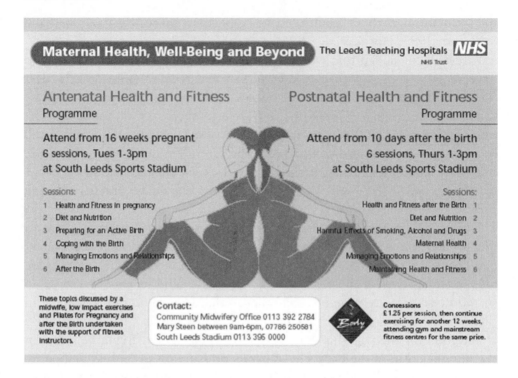

FIGURE 7.3 Maternal health, well-being and beyond.

> I'm going to be as active as possible in labour.
> I found using the birth ball really helpful.
> I'm definitely going to be active and use the positions I have been taught.
> I can't believe I can have a homebirth if I want.

Promoting active birth

Being able to move around during labour has been identified as a vital component for labour to progress (Gould, 2000). In her own home, a woman can move around freely and use a variety of furniture and props that help her to adopt different postures and positions (Albers, 2007). She will naturally use lots of different postures and positions during the birth process (Gardosi *et al.*, 1989). It has been recommended by the National Institute for Health and Clinical Excellence (2007) that women should be encouraged and helped to move and adopt whatever positions they find most comfortable throughout labour. The homebirth environment is ideal for the woman to have an active birth as it encourages and enables her to move around freely. The midwife is in an optimum position to encourage this and mobilisation is associated with a reduction in complications caused by restricted movement and semirecumbent postures (Gupta *et al.*, 2004).

First stage of labour

Ideally women should be encouraged to adopt upright positions during the first stage of labour as there are significant advantages to assuming an upright position in labour and birth. These include gravity, reduced risk of aortocaval compression, better alignment of the fetus, more efficient contractions and increased pelvic outlet in squatting and kneeling positions (MIDIRS, 2005). Use of postural coping strategies during the first stage of labour is associated with providing some pain relief and helping a woman to cope with pain (Spiby *et al*., 2003; Simkin and Bolding 2004). A clinical trial has reported no harmful effects have been associated with walking during labour, and women should be encouraged to do this if they wish (Bloom *et al*., 1998).

A variety of positions can assist women in the first stage of labour to progress and cope. Changing positions in the first stage leads to effective contractions (Gupta and Nikodem, 2001) and leaning forward is particularly helpful for women who have a baby in an OP position. Many women find sitting astride a chair (Figure 7.4) and even sitting on the toilet comfortable. Some women

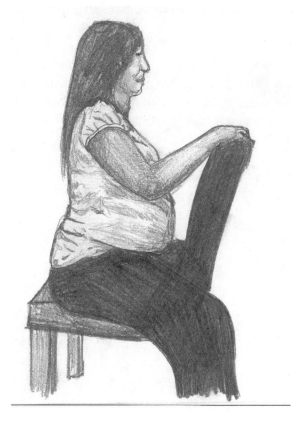

FIGURE 7.4 Woman astride a chair.

put a pillow upon a table or the cistern and have a short catnap. Some women obtain relief from pelvic rocking, and a birth ball, rocking chair or beanbag are useful props to promote movement and being active.

Second stage of labour

Upright positions should also be encouraged in the second stage of labour. These include sitting (more than 45° from the horizontal), squatting or kneeling, or crouching on all fours (Figure 7.5). A Cochrane review concluded that the adopting an upright position during the second stage of labour has many benefits, including a reduction in the duration of the second stage and a reduction in the number instrumental births and episiotomies, although estimated blood loss was reported to be greater (Gupta *et al.*, 2004). It has been reported that adopting a lateral position for birth appears to protect the perineum (Shorten *et al.*, 2002). However, squatting using a birthing chair has been reported to be a predisposing factor for third and fourth degree tears (Jander and Lyrenas, 2001).

A variety of positions can assist women in the second stage of labour to progress and cope. It is advisable to demonstrate these antenatally and for the woman to practise.

'Squatting' or being in a 'knees and leaning forward' position has the advantage of increasing the pelvic outlet. The pelvic outlet is 1 cm greater in the transverse diameter and 2 cm greater in the anteroposterior diameter, resulting in an increase in the pelvic outlet area of approximately 28 per cent when compared with a supine position (Russell, 1982). However, many women are

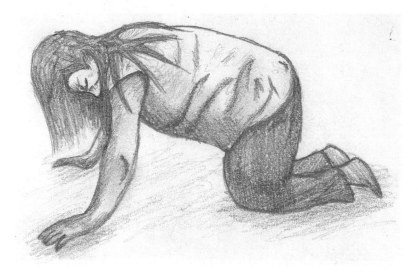

FIGURE 7.5 Woman on all fours.

not able to squat comfortably and find the 'knees and leaning forward position' more comfortable. Some women opt for the squatting position and get their partners to support and hold them up. Just as in the first stage of labour, upright positions are gravity assisted and some women will prefer to adopt a high sitting position, be semirecumbent, kneel or squat on a birthing cushion to assist them to give birth.

Birth balls

The use of birth balls is gaining in popularity and they are not too expensive to purchase. Midwives can recommend 'gym balls', which may be slightly cheaper in cost and are basically of a similar design. These balls can be used during pregnancy and are particularly helpful for women who are suffering from backache and suprapubic pain. Sitting on one of these balls encourages women to sit upright, and this will align the neutral curves in their vertebrae. Women can practise pelvic rocking and adopting different positions that they may find helpful when labour commences. During labour, many women find leaning forward and using the ball like a big cushion comfortable (Figure 7.6), and often this induces a 'catnap' between contractions and helps women to reserve some energy. Women can also remain in an upright, squatting position, and this maximises their pelvic outlet. Rocking the pelvis from side to side and backwards and forwards while sitting on a birth ball (Figure 7.7) has been reported to ease pain and discomfort felt during the first and second stages of labour (Watkins, 2001). Birth balls appear to help women focus on

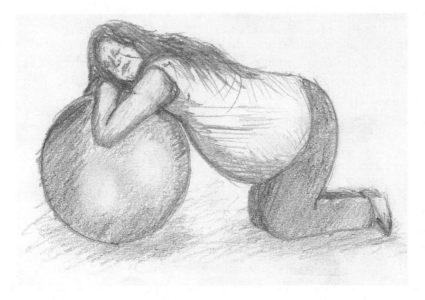

FIGURE 7.6 Woman using a birth ball as a big cushion.

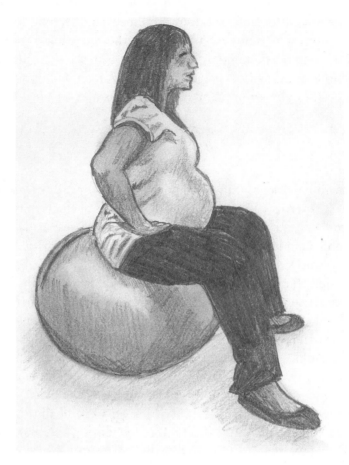

FIGURE 7.7 Woman sitting on a birth ball.

working with their labour pains and will be a useful aid to have available for a homebirth. In addition, following the birth, there are several toning exercises that can be carried out using one of these balls, and this will assist a woman to return back to her non-pregnant body shape, increasing her self-esteem and well-being.

Breathing exercises

Lamaze (1958) recognised the benefit of teaching a woman breathing exercises during childbirth as a natural way to help her remain calm and relaxed. Teaching women how to breathe slowly and steadily during pregnancy will help them to achieve this in labour and for birth. It will help women to remain calm and can also help their partner or alternative birth partner too. During antenatal education classes, breathing exercises to assist a woman and her partner to stay focused and calm during labour are taught. For example, breathing in for the count of 5 and out for the count of 7 will slow a woman's breathing, respirations and heart rate. It will help a woman to relax and stop her panicking. During labour, a woman's breathing rhythms will naturally increase when she is having a contraction, and this may make her feel a little anxious. When a woman starts to feel a contraction commencing she can also instinctively hold her breath and forget to breathe. It is important for the woman to concentrate and remember to breathe throughout the duration of her contraction as this will help her to get oxygen into her lungs and aid coping. A midwife and the woman's partner can play an important role here and remind the woman to breathe when she feels a contraction starting.

Relaxation techniques

Music and meditation CDs are also a soothing and comforting way to help women relax during labour. A good idea is to advise women and their partner to put their favourite tunes on to a CD or an iPod, as this will help both of them to relax and reduce their fear. Often women like to hum or count to the beat of a favourite tune during a contraction as this helps them stay focused and positive. Listening to a meditation CD can also produce a state of self-hypnosis and help women stay focused and calm. Relaxation techniques can help reduce the severity of pain experienced by a woman in labour and help her cope (Lamaze, 1958).

Meditation can promote a spiritual connection during labour. Many women have described their experiences of childbirth as being associated with a spiritual uplifting (Dick-Read, 1959). Music and meditation can enhance this aspect of childbirth and promote a positive birth experience.

Self-hypnosis

Hypnotherapy involves inducing a state of concentration which, when combined with relaxation techniques, allows a heightened state of awareness caused by suggestion. The use during labour of self-hypnosis, which is guided by visualising, imagery and breathing techniques to utilise natural hormones and induce a state of deep relaxed concentration, is known as hypnobirthing and is becoming an increasingly popular natural method for women to use. This natural method is based on 'the fear–tension–pain' syndrome of childbirth first described by the famous English physician Grantly Dick-Read, who believed that when fear is eliminated most women are then able to birth naturally (see Chapter 4). Women are still fully aware of what is happening around them and this method can make them feel like they are day-dreaming or drifting off to sleep. Self-hypnosis appears to help women be less anxious and frightened during labour, and this in turn helps them to cope with labour pain. The woman's partner can help her use some hypnotic techniques, and both of them can attend classes from about 25–30 weeks of pregnancy to learn how to do it and practise the techniques before the woman goes into labour. Some midwives have undertaken further training to assist them to help women to learn self-hypnosis techniques. Many women who opt for a homebirth will consider this option and midwives need to find out where women can access classes locally.

Hypnobirthing techniques are a good way to promote normal birth, and there is evidence that this method has the potential to reduce the length of labour and the need for medical intervention (Jenkins and Pritchard, 1993; Hao and Li, 1997; Martin *et al.*, 2001).

Massage

Many women find being touched during labour helpful; it can reduce fear, anxiety, tension and pain. For example, the touch of someone who cares about the woman and wants to help and support her during labour has been shown to promote normal birth. Massaging the woman during labour will stimulate her body to release endorphins, which are natural pain-killing and mood-lifting substances. Gentle massage and slight pressure can also stimulate contractions when they are not coordinated. Birth partners can be taught how to massage their partners in labour. An antenatal massage programme in which midwives and birth partners are taught specific massage techniques for supporting women during labour has had positive results (McNabb *et al.*, 2006). Another study found that women who were massaged during labour were less anxious and experienced less pain as well and had shorter labours and less postnatal depression than a control group of women who were not massaged (Simkin and O'Hara, 2002).

There is some evidence that teaching massage and relaxation techniques to fathers to assist during labour (Figure 7.8) is an effective way to increase marital satisfaction and decrease postnatal depressive symptoms (Latifses *et al.*, 2005). Massage also provides psychosocial support for women (M.Y. Chang *et al.*, 2002).

Many women and their birth partners find using massage very helpful during labour. Massage involves touch techniques which induce relaxation, a sense of well-being and alleviate labour pain. A birth partner will also find massage relaxing and therapeutic. Ideally, when attending antenatal classes, a birth partner will have had an opportunity to observe a midwife demonstrating some techniques and the chance to practise some of them.

General points about massage:

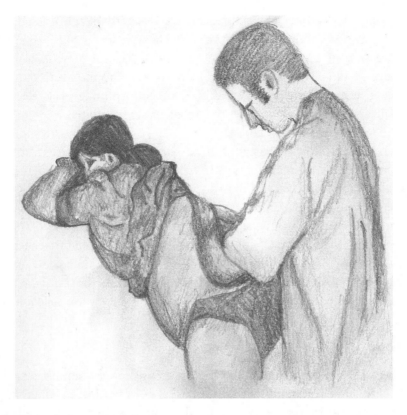

Figure 7.8 The father massaging.

- It conveys a message of support and care.
- It gives a message of understanding and encouragement.
- However, not all women will want to be touched.
- The massager needs to be alert to cues, and aware of when and when not to massage.
- A midwife should teach birth partners how to, and when.

Using a variety of massage movements to the head, neck, shoulders and lower back is particularly helpful to relieve stress, tension and fatigue felt in labour.

Acupressure

Acupressure involves therapeutic touch, and it can be helpful to induce labour and relieve pain in early labour (Betts, 2006). Acupressure therapy has been used for centuries by the Chinese and is believed to help open the channels of energy and increases blood circulation to nourish the main organs, glands, muscles, nerves and vital centres of the body (S.T. Chang, 1995).

Acupressure techniques can increase the levels of endorphins, which help to reduce fear and anxiety. Acupressure can also foster a sense of spirituality. Acupressure involves massage and the application of pressure to specific acupressure points (the same points as used in acupuncture) to induce a deeply relaxing experience which will increase endorphin levels (Betts, 2006). Acupressure therapy is effective in the relief of stress-related ailments and is therefore ideal for women in labour.

Shiatsu (a well-known style of acupressure) is a method that stimulates acupressure points and meridians to relieve stress, tension and pain. It is a traditional therapeutic form of massage that uses firm pressure to stimulate acupressure points. A shiatsu practitioner can use different parts of her hand, that is, fingers, thumbs, palms, side of her hand or her knuckles, to apply firm pressure (Yates, 2003). Some local areas now have complementary therapy centres with a shiatsu or acupressure practitioner available. Women can access one of these practitioners if they want to try this option. *Shiatsu for Midwives* (Yates, 2003) is an excellent resource for midwives to read if they want to learn more.

Reflexology

Reflexology involves massaging the 'reflex zones' on a woman's feet, hands and also ears that correspond with different parts of her body to help improve her blood circulation and relax any tension she maybe feeling. Reflexology is gaining some popularity during pregnancy and labour. Some maternity units in the UK are now offering reflexology as a therapy. Women may have reflexology to help them relax during pregnancy and labour. Some women have reported that reflexology has assisted them go into labour when they are overdue (Leino, 2011). Reflexology is based on certain reflex areas on the feet and hands that directly affect the main organs and muscles of the woman's body. It is similar to acupressure as it applies pressure to specific points on the body. However, reflexology does not work with the body's energy flow in the same way as acupressure.

This method may be comforting for some women but not all. Many women naturally want to be active and moving around during their labour so this may be more helpful for women during early labour, in between contractions, but less so as labour progresses. *Reflexology in Pregnancy and Childbirth*, a recent book by Denise Tiran, provides a useful guide and helpful information (Tiran, 2010).

Acupuncture

The use of acupuncture in pregnancy, during childbirth and following birth is also gaining some popularity in the UK. Sarah Budd was one of the first midwives to establish an acupuncture clinic in a maternity unit (Budd, 2000). Sue Ng, a midwife/acupuncturist based in the north of England, is presently running a very successful acupuncture clinic.

A recent systematic review and meta-analysis that included 10 randomised controlled trials reported limited evidence to confirm whether acupuncture can control pain during established labour when compared with no pain relief, conventional analgesia, a placebo or sham acupuncture (Cho *et al.*, 2010). However, the researchers did report that women were less likely to use other forms of analgesia and acknowledged that the heterogeneity of the studies (large variation in the results from one study to the other) made interpretation difficult. Pain is a syndrome in its own right and extremely complex to measure; the trials included in this meta-analysis focused on the intensity of pain, which is only one dimension of the pain experience. The quality of pain and individuals' perceptions need to be taken into consideration. There is no evidence of harm to the mother or her baby from the use of acupuncture in labour and this is an option that some women may want to consider. For further information read *Essential Guide to Acupuncture in Pregnancy and Childbirth* by Debra Betts (2006). This book is easy to read and includes practical and useful information on how acupuncture can help some women cope with labour.

Aromatherapy

Aromatherapy (essential) oils are derived from plants and used to promote health and well-being and also for their therapeutic properties in many conditions. Many women are now using these oils during their pregnancy, childbirth experience and following birth (Mitchell *et al.*, 2006). Some women having a homebirth will opt to use aromatherapy, and it has been reported that both women and midwives find the use of aromatherapy in labour to be beneficial (Burns *et al.*, 1999, 2000). There are aromatherapy birth kits that the woman can purchase, but it is advisable that the woman consults a qualified aromatherapist to discuss what essential oils are beneficial and safe to use during pregnancy and labour. Some are contraindicated in pregnancy and only oils known to be safe in pregnancy and labour should be used (Tiran, 2000). For example, the essential oil clary sage is not recommended during pregnancy as it can stimulate tightenings; however, it is commonly used during labour to help relieve stress and tension and lift a woman's spirits, although it contraindicated if the woman is using Entonox. Continuous vaporisation may have adverse maternal effects, in particular clouding concentration (Tiran, 2006).

The use of aromatherapy oils during childbirth can stimulate, refresh and soothe labouring women and to some extent can also assist their partner and the midwife in attendance to remain calm and relaxed. During childbirth aromatherapy oils can be helpful to alleviate stress, and there is some evidence that aromatherapy oils can reduce anxiety and fear during labour, which in turn helps a woman cope with labour pain (Burns *et al.*, 2000).

Essential oils can be can be utilised in several ways during labour and birth. A woman can have an aromatic bath during labour and following birth to help her relax. An oil burner or vaporiser can scent the room, helping to create a calm, relaxing atmosphere. A blend of oils, for example lavender, clary sage and jasmine, in a carrier oil such as almond oil, jojoba oil, grapeseed, olive oil or wheatgerm can be massaged directly into the skin on the shoulders, back, legs, feet and hands. Hot and cold compresses with essential oils added to the water prior to the compress being rung out and used as a wet cloth can also be very soothing during contractions and following contractions. A facial spritz combining water and essential oils and stored in the fridge can refresh a woman in established labour.

The following essential oils may be helpful to a woman in labour:

- *Bergamot*. Has a refreshing and uplifting effect.
- *Chamomile*. Has a soothing and calming effect to reduce anxiety.
- *Clary sage*. Can strengthen contractions during labour, reduce anxiety and lift a woman's spirits (not recommended when Entonox is being used).
- *Geranium*. Helps breathing and circulation.
- *Jasmine*. Relieves pain and acts as a uterine tonic and an antispasmodic.
- *Lavender*. Has a relaxing and calming effect and relieves anxiety, tension and pain.
- *Marjoram*. Has uterine tonic, pain-relieving, antispasmodic properties and can also help with breathing to lower blood pressure.
- *Neroli*. Has antidepressant, calming and relaxing effects.
- *Rose*. Has uterine tonic and antidepressant affects.

The cost of these essential oils can vary and this needs to be taken into consideration. For example, lavender oil is relatively inexpensive when compared with rose oil. A book entitled *Clinical Aromatherapy for Pregnancy and Childbirth* is a good resource for midwives who want to learn more (Tiran, 2000).

Homeopathy

Homeopathy is based on a principle known as the 'law of similars', which states that a substance that can cause symptoms when given to healthy people can help to heal those who are suffering from similar symptoms. For example, a homeopathic preparation made from coffee can relieve insomnia.

Homeopathic remedies are used to treat a wide range of conditions and are different from herbal medicines as they are diluted and then potentised (Steen and Calvert, 2006).

There are several remedies that can be helpful for a woman to take during her labour and childbirth. Women can self-administer these, and there are several childbirth kits available for her to purchase. The kits contain ampoules of different potentised remedies, each of has been diluted and succussed 30 times, and a guide to which remedy to take depending on symptoms (Calvert and Steen, 2007). To administer the remedy, a drop is applied to a sucrose tablet and the tablet sucked. In this way, the remedy is absorbed through the mucous membrane of the mouth, rather than the digestive system, and so can be effective even when someone is vomiting (Steen and Calvert, 2007).

The most common remedies include:

- aconite: for fear;
- arnica: the healer;
- calendula: wound mender;
- caulophyllum: uterine tonic;
- chamomilla: for pain;
- gelsemium: to relieve anxiety;
- kali carbonicum: for backache;
- kali phosphoricum: for exhaustion;
- nux vomica: one for dad;
- pulsatilla: for the weak and weepy.
- *Aconite*. A woman can take aconite if she is panicky and full of fear. A woman needing aconite is restless – her partner may need it as well if he is pacing around anxiously! If the labour is very hard or fast and the woman is shell-shocked afterwards and cannot pass urine, then aconite may help.
- *Arnica*. Arnica is good for keeping a woman going during a tiring labour and helping to relieve pain. A woman can take 30 ml of arnica every hour once the labour is established. She can also take arnica after the birth to help her heal and it is also helpful for afterpains.
- *Calendula*. Calendula may help a woman heal if she has a perineal tear, episiotomy or caesarean section wound.
- *Caulophyllum*. Caulophyllum is useful if a woman's labour does not progress or stops, or she has labour pains which are not effective and her cervix is not dilating. She may be thirsty, shivery and tired.
- *Chamomilla*. If a woman cannot stand the pain any more and just wants drugs or a caesarean, try chamomilla. The woman may be showing signs of anger, impatience or becoming abusive because the pain feels unbearable.

- *Gelsemium*. This remedy may help a woman if she feels very anxious leading up to giving birth. She may be shivery, nervous, have visual disturbances and feel scared stiff!
- *Kali carbonicum*. This is for a backache labour or if a woman's baby is lying in a posterior position. A woman can take this remedy as needed, every five minutes if necessary, to get her through.
- *Kali phosphoricum*. This remedy is for exhaustion and can be administered between contractions until some energy is restored.
- *Nux vomica*. A remedy for birth partners who think they might faint or cannot cope with the sight of blood.
- *Pulsatilla*. If a woman feels weepy and clingy and cannot go on, then this remedy can help. A woman can also use this remedy after birth if she get 'the blues' in the week following the birth.

Childbirth requires a lot of energy, so remedies may need to be repeated quickly and regularly to stimulate a response and the partner can support you here. Women will need different remedies as their labour progresses. Alternatively, a woman can consult a registered homeopath, who will prescribe her remedies based on her individual symptom picture taking into account her mental, emotional and physical needs (Steen and Calvert, 2006).

Homeopathic remedies have been used to help women through many experiences of pregnancy and childbirth. There has, however, been very little research in this area to date. The author of this chapter and editor of this book (Mary Steen) has been involved in some qualitative research to explore women's views and experiences on the use of a homeopathic childbirth remedies kit. Nineteen women were asked to complete a semistructured questionnaire that asked questions relating to their knowledge about and use of homeopathy and to elicit the reasons why and when the respondents decided to take a remedy, which remedy they chose and their perceived response to the remedy. A semistructured interview technique was used to follow up these women after the birth. Women reported that they had gained positive benefits from using the kit of homeopathic remedies. Some birth partners also used some remedies to alleviate nausea, tiredness, anxiety, fear and anger. Some women reported that the kit also had a positive impact on their birth partner, enabling them to provide calm and confident support during labour. Four general themes were generated from the interviews: how remedies were used; empowerment; emotional needs; and dads and birth partners. The final core theme identified was a positive birth experience regardless of the mode of delivery. The interviews demonstrated that women and several birth partners experienced positive emotional, psychological and physical benefits from using the kit of homeopathic remedies (Steen and Calvert, 2006, 2007; Calvert and Steen, 2007).

Water

Women throughout history have used hydrotherapy to help ease labour pains, and some have given birth in shallow water, for example, women living in the South Pacific. In the 1970s, Michael Odent, a French obstetrician, reintroduced the concept of waterbirth to the Western world, and it has become an increasingly popular method to use for labour and birth. It is not uncommon for birth centres to offer the option of a waterbirth, but not all maternity units offer this choice. However, in a woman's own home this choice is freely available. Hydrotherapy is an excellent way to alleviate aches and pains and promote relaxation. It is used in many painful conditions, and choosing to have a waterbirth at home can be a helpful way for women to cope with labour pains and childbirth. However, at present there is limited research evidence to confirm or refute the benefits of actual birth in water. There appears to be no difference in the length of labour or the baby's Apgar scores. However, anecdotally, women's experiences tend to suggest that less analgesia is required, they feel more relaxed and have less backache and the likelihood of perineal tears is reduced. Postpartum haemorrhage is rare and most women will opt for a physiological third stage. There is no evidence to support the theoretical risk that a woman or her baby is at increased risk of an infection, and there are no recorded cases of water embolism (Confidential Enquiry into Maternal and Child Health, 2004).

Many women find being in a warm water bath during labour and then giving birth in water to be very soothing and an excellent way to cope with labour pains. Often, a slow labour can improve when a woman immerses herself in a birth pool and starts to relax. Over the last decade or so, this natural method has become more commonly available for women and many women opt for a waterbirth in their home (Figure 7.9). All midwives should be able to support and assist a woman who chooses to have a waterbirth. Midwives need to know where women can hire a mobile waterbirth pool and single-use liner if they decide to opt for this method. Ideally, a 'trial run' of filling the pool and trying it out in the antenatal period is recommended. The National Institute for Health and Clinical Excellence (2007) recommends that the temperature of the water should be approximately 37–37.5°C (body temperature). It is important during the woman's labour to continuously monitor the water temperature and maintain the recommended temperature. Ideally, have plenty of towels available to use and a bowl to collect any faeces.

A small stool or even sitting on a birth ball can be a valuable aid for a midwife when supporting a woman who has opted for a waterbirth. During the woman's labour, a midwife can sit adjacent to the pool and keep in close contact with the woman. Women may also opt to use other pain management

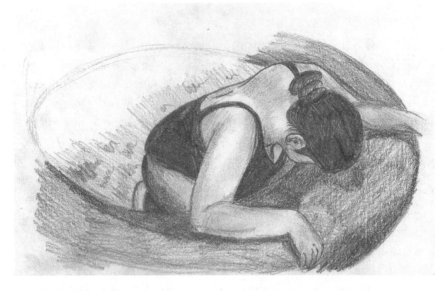

FIGURE 7.9 Woman and waterbirth.

methods, such as portable Entonox, whilst in the pool as labour progresses. (See case study 6 in Chapter 8, 'Homebirth – waterbirth'.)

Transcutaneous electrical nerve stimulation

Transcutaneous electrical nerve stimulation (TENS) stimulates a woman's body's to produce enkephalins and endorphins, which are her natural pain-killers. TENS also reduces pain signals sent to her brain by the spinal cord. It can be used at the end of pregnancy (after 36 weeks) if a woman has any backache or if the Braxton Hicks contractions are becoming uncomfortable for her to cope with.

Four electrodes are taped to the lower back and connected by wires to a small battery-operated stimulator (box), known as an 'obstetric pulsar', which the woman can hold or have near her during labour. The woman needs to be advised on how to use this and be advised to turn the TENS on at a low-intensity setting, which she can gradually increase as a way to cope with the intensity of her labour pains. Some TENS machines have a booster facility so she can give herself an extra boost if her contractions are getting stronger. There are no known side-effects for either the woman or her baby and the labouring woman can still be active and move around while using this method (Mainstone, 2004).

The National Institute for Health and Clinical Excellence (2007) has controversially and without substantial evidence recommended that TENS should not be used in established labour. Despite conflicting opinions on its

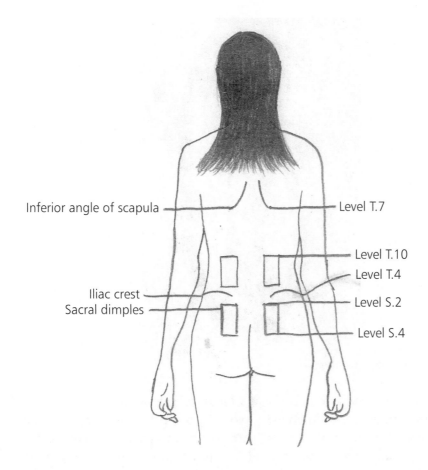

Inferior angle of scapula — Level T.7

Level T.10
Level T.4

Iliac crest
Sacral dimples — Level S.2

Level S.4

Figure 7.10 A woman using a TENS machine.

effectiveness, including the possibility of a placebo effect, TENS is reported by many women to provide effective pain relief, especially in the first stage of labour (Johnson, 1997). (See case study 1 in Chapter 8, 'Homebirth – no complications'.)

Entonox

Entonox is possibly the most common analgesia used in labour in the UK (Charles, 2009). The use of a mixture of 50 per cent nitrous oxide and 50 per cent oxygen in one cylinder for the relief of pain in childbirth was researched and introduced to maternity services approximately 50 years ago by Tunstall (1961). Its effects are short-lasting as it is rapidly excreted from the system. It is an inhaled form of pain relief that women can easily use in their own home. It is exhaled very quickly and it has no known side-effects on the fetus. In fact, it can improve fetal oxygenation. Its effect is relatively rapid and it

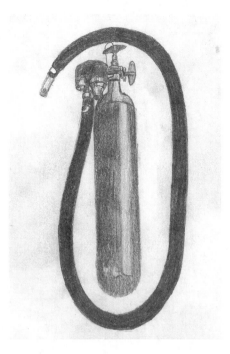

Figure 7.11 The Entonox cylinder.

takes approximately one minute for a woman to gain some pain relief. For this reason a midwife should advise a woman to start inhaling at the beginning of a contraction, so that feels the effect at the peak of a contraction. Between contractions a woman should be advised to stop inhaling. Entonox is self-administered via a demand valve using a mouthpiece and can be used in association with other analgesia. A woman may complain of a dry mouth when inhaling Entonox and she should be advised to take frequent sips of water or ice to crunch. Entonox can make a women feel dizzy, a bit disorientated and nauseous, so a woman should be made aware of this and advised to breathe normally between contractions. During childbirth, a woman's movements can be restricted when inhaling Entonox, but she can remain in an upright position up until giving birth and it will not affect her urge to push in the second stage. The Entonox cylinder needs to be used at room temperature for effective administration, and a midwife needs to ensure that health and safety measures are adhered to (BOC, 2010). (See case study 2 in Chapter 8, 'Homebirth – need to transfer-in to consultant-led unit.)

Analgesia

Pethidine, diamorphine and Meptid are occasionally used by women as analgesia during a homebirth when they perceive the pain to be severe. Pethidine appears to be the opiate most commonly used at a homebirth. In some cases, although it is prescribed, it is not actually used, but 'knowing' it is available if needed seems to give some women reassurance. If it is not used, then it is the woman's responsibility to return the ampoule to the pharmacist or dispose of the contents. A midwife can supervise this.

Opiates are the strongest form of analgesia available to use during a homebirth. They are given intramuscularly and take about 15–20 minutes to have an effect. The effects usually last for approximately two to four hours. Some women find that this form of pain relief helps and allows them time to rest. However, it is associated with maternal, fetal and neonatal side-effects. The maternal effects are nausea and vomiting and hypotension (Elbourne and Wiseman, 2006), disorientation and a feeling of loss of control; the progress of labour may be slowed (Charles, 2009). An antiemetic should be given simultaneously as a prophylactic for nausea and vomiting (National Institute for Health and Clinical Excellence, 2007). Neonatal side-effects include respiratory depression and subdued behaviour patterns, such as a diminished response to sight and sounds, drowsiness and a reluctance to feed, which may impair early breast-feeding (Elbourne and Wiseman, 2006; National Institute for Health and Clinical Excellence, 2007). An antidote (naloxone, 400μg in 1 ml) can be administered intramuscularly to the baby as soon as he/she is born if these side-effects are present. The mother must be made aware that these side-effects may last for several days in the baby and may interfere with breast-feeding.

Conclusions

Women need to be aware of their choice to have a homebirth and what care and support they will receive. They need to be well prepared and have a good knowledge of ways to work with the pain and the pain management options that are available for them to adopt and use. A familiar, safe homely environment can help a woman to remain calm and relaxed and to progress in labour. Companionship and support are essential components to promote a normal birth within the home. Remaining active during labour and using a range of different positions in labour has been shown to be beneficial to women and will shorten the length of labour.

Alternative and complementary therapies can play an important part in meeting the woman's physical, emotional, psychological and spiritual needs during childbirth. At home there will be no restrictions in using one or several of these therapies to assist a woman during her childbirth experience. In addition, inhalation and injected analgesia methods are available upon a woman's request but is important that the woman is fully aware of any side-effects associated with these methods and makes an informed decision based on her individual needs.

References

Betts, D. (2006) *Essential Guide to Acupuncture in Pregnancy & Childbirth*. Hove: Journal of Chinese Medicine.

Bloom, S.L., McIntire, D.D., Kelly, M.A., Beimer, H.L., Burpo, R.H., Garcia, M.A. and Leveno, K.J. (1998) Lack of effect of walking on labor and delivery. *New England Journal of Medicine*, 339, 76–9.

Bonica, J.J. (1994) Labour pain. In Wall, P.D. and Melzack, R. (eds.) *Textbook of Pain*. New York: Churchill Livingstone, pp. 377–92.

Brayshaw, E. (2003) *Exercise for Pregnancy and Childbirth: A Practical Guide for Educators*. Oxford: Books for Midwives.

British Oxygen Company (2010) Entonox (http://www.boconline.co.uk/products/products_by_industry/emergency-services; accessed 26 January 2011).

Brooke, E. (1997) *Medicine Women: A Pictorial History of Women Healers*. Wheaton, IL: Quest Books.

Budd, A. (2000) Acupuncture. In Tiran, D. and Mack, S. (eds.) *Complementary Therapies of Pregnancy and Childbirth*. London: Baillière Tindall.

Burns E., Blamey, C., Ersser, S.J., Lloyd, A.J. and Barnetson, L. (1999) *The Use of Aromatherapy in Intrapartum Midwifery Practice. An Evaluative Study*. Oxford: Oxford Centre of Health Care Research & Development, Oxford Brookes University.

Butler, C.L., Williams, M.A., Sorensen, T.K., Frederick, I.O. and Leisenring, W.M. (2004) Relation between maternal recreational physical activity and plasma lipids in early pregnancy. *American Journal of Epidemiology*, 160, 350–9.

Calvert, J. and Steen, M. (2007) Homeopathic remedies for self-administration during childbirth. *British Journal of Midwifery*, 15, 159–65.

Chang, M.Y., Wang, S.Y. and Chen, C.H. (2002) Effects of massage on pain and anxiety during labour: a randomised controlled trial in Taiwan. *Journal of Advanced Nursing*, 38, 68–73.

Chang, S.T. (1995) *The Complete Book of Acupuncture*. Berkeley, CA: Celestial Arts.

Cho, S.-H., Lee, H. and Ernst, E. (2010) Acupuncture for pain relief in labour: a systematic review and meta-analysis. *BJOG* (DOI 10.1111/j.1471–0528.2010.02570.x).

Clapp, J.F. (2001) Recommending exercise during pregnancy. *Journal of Paediatrics, Obstetrics and Gynaecology*, 27(4), 21–8.

Confidential Enquiry into Maternal and Child Health (CEMACH) (2004) *Why Mothers Die, 2000 to 2002*. London: Royal College of Obstetricians and Gynaecologists.

Department of Health (2004) *National Service Framework for Children, Young People and Maternity Services*. Standard 11: Maternity Services. London: Department of Health.

Dick-Read, G. (1959) Childbirth in emergency. In *Childbirth without Fear: The Principles and Practices of Natural Childbirth*, 4th edn. London: Heinemann Medical Books.

Donnison, J. (1988) *Midwives and Medicine Men: A History of the Struggle for the Control of Childbirth*, 2nd edn. New Barnett, UK: Historical Publications.

Downe, S. (2004) *Normal Birth Evidence and Debate*. Edinburgh: Churchill Livingstone.

Elbourne, D. and Wiseman, R.R.E.W. (2006) Types of intra-muscular opioids for maternal pain relief in labour. *Cochrane Database of Systematic Reviews*, Issue 2, article no. CD001237 (DOI 10.1002/14651858.CD001237.pub2).

Ernst, E., Schmidt, K. and Wider, B. (2005) CAM research in Britain: the last 10 years. *Complementary Therapies in Clinical Medicine*, 11, 17–20,

Friederickson, R. and Geary, L.E. (1982) Endogenous opioids peptides, review of physiological, pharmacological and clinical aspects. *Programmes in Neurobiology*, 19, 19–69.

Frye, A. (2004) Anatomy and physiology of uterine changes during late pregnancy and labor. In *Holistic Midwifery: A Comprehensive Textbook for Midwives in Homebirth Practice. Vol. II: Care of the Mother and Baby from the Onset of Labor through the First Hours after Birth.* Oregon: Labrys Press, pp. 256–2.

Gaskin, I.M. (2008) *Ina May's Guide to Childbirth.* London: Vermilion.

Goldstein, A. (1978) Endorphins. *Science*, 18, 14–19.

Gupta, J.K., Hofmeyr, G.J. and Smyth, R. (2004) Position in the second stage of labour for women without epidural anaesthesia. *Cochrane Database of Systematic Reviews*, issue 1, article no. CD002006 (DOI 10.1002/14651858.CD002006.pub2).

Hao, T.Y., Li, Y.H. and Yao, S.F. (1997) Clinical study on shortening the birth process using psychological suggestion therapy. *Zhonghua Hu Li Za Zhi*, 32, 568–70.

Hodnett, E.D., Gates, S., Hofymer, G.J., Sakala, C. and Weston, J. (2011) Continuous support during childbirth. *Cochrane Database of Systematic Reviews*, Issue 2, article no. CD003766 (DOI 10.1002/14651858.CD003766.pub3).

Horns, P., Ratcliffe, L., Leggett, J. and Swanson, M. (1996) Pregnancy outcomes among active and sedentary primiparous women. *Journal of Obstetric, Gynaecological and Neonatal Nursing Clinical Studies*, 25(1), 49–54.

Hughes, J., Smith, T.W., Kosterlitz, H.W. and Fothergill, L.A. (1975) Identification of two related peptides from the brain with potent agonist activity. *Nature*, 258, 577–9.

Jander, C. and Lyrenas, S, (2001) Third and fourth degree perineal tears. Predictor factors in a referral hospital. *Acta Obstetrica et Gynecologica Scandinavica*, 80, 229–34.

Jenkins, M.W. and Pritchard, M.H (1993) Hypnosis: applications and theoretical considerations in normal labour. *British Journal of Obstetrics and Gynaecology*, 100, 221–6.

Johnson, M.I. (1997) Transcutaneous electrical nerve stimulation (TENS) in the management of labour pain: the experience of over ten thousand women. *British Journal of Midwifery*, 5, 400–5.

Johnson, M.I. (2006) Physiology of pain. In White, R. and Harding, K. (eds.) *Trauma and Pain in Wound Management.* Aberdeen: Wounds UK publications, pp. 17–58.

Kramer, M.S. and McDonald, S.W. (2006) Aerobic exercise for women during pregnancy. *Cochrane Database of Systematic Reviews*, Issue 3, Article No. CD000180 (DOI 10.1002/14651858.CD000180.pub2).

Lamaze, F. (1958) *Painless Childbirth: Psychoprophylactic Method.* London: Burke.

Latifses, V., Bendell Estroff, D., Field, T. and Bush, J.P (2005) Fathers massaging and relaxing their pregnant wives lowered anxiety and facilitated marital adjustment. *Journal of Bodywork and Movement Therapies*, 9, 277–82.

Leino, L. (2011) Maternity acupressure: how to induce labor and have an easier, safer and shorter birth (http://www.maternityacupressure.com/index.html; accessed 17 March 2011).

McNabb, M., Kimbler, L., Haines, A. and McCourt, C. (2006) Does regular massage from late pregnancy to birth decrease maternal pain perception during labour and birth? A feasibility study to investigate a programme of massage, controlled breathing and visualization from 36 weeks of pregnancy until birth. *Complementary Therapies in Clinical Practice*, 12, 222–31.

Mainstone, A. (2004) TENS. *British Journal of Midwifery*, 12, 578–81.

Martin, A.A., Schauble, P.G., Surekha, H.R. and Curry, Jr, R.W. (2001) The effects of hypnosis on the labor processes and birth outcomes of pregnant adolescents. *Journal of Family Practice*, 50, 441–3.

Melzack, R. and Wall, P.D. (1965) Pain mechanisms: a new theory. *Science*, 150, 971–9.

Melzack, R. and Wall, P.D. (1996) The theories of pain. In *The Challenge of Pain.* London: Penguin Books, pp. 147–65.

Mitchell, M. and Williams, J. (2007) The role of midwife-complementary therapists: data from in-depth interviews. *Evidence Based Midwifery*, 5(3), 93–9

Mitchell, M., Williams, J., Hobbs, E. and Pollard, K. (2006) The use of complementary therapies in maternity services: a survey. *British Journal of Midwifery*, 14, 576–82.

National Institute for Health and Clinical Excellence (2007) *Intrapartum Care*. Clinical Guideline 55. London: National Institute for Health and Clinical Excellence.

NMC (2004) *Midwives' Rules and Standards*. London: NMC (http://www.nmc-uk.org/aFrameDisplay.aspx?DocumentID=169; accessed 28 February 2011).

NMC (2006a) *Complementary Therapies and Homeopathy*. London: NMC (http://www.nmc-uk.org/aFrameDisplay.aspx?DocumentID=1559; accessed 28 February 2011).

NMC (2006b) *Medicine Management*. London: NMC (http://www.nmc-uk.org/aFrameDisplay.aspx?DocumentID=1801; accessed 28 February 2011).

O'Hara, P. (1996) *Pain Management for Health Professionals*. London: Chapman & Hall.

Raouf, R., Quick, K. and Wood, J.N. (2010) Visceral pain: pain as a channelopathy. *Journal Clinical Investigation*, 120, 3745–52.

Rice, A.S.C. (1992) Pain, inflammation and wound healing. In: Proceedings of the 3rd European Conference on Advances in Wound Management, Harrogate, UK.

Royal College of Midwives (2005) Campaign for Normal Birth. London: Royal College of Midwives (www.rcmnormalbirth.org.org.uk; accessed 28 February 2011).

Royal College of Midwives (2007) *Complementary and Alternative Therapies*. Guidance Paper No. 6. Fyle, J, and Steen, M. (eds.). London: Royal College of Midwives.

Royal College of Midwives (2008) *Evidence Based Guidelines for Midwifery-Led Care in Labour*. Jokinen, M. and Munro, J. (eds.). London: Royal College of Midwives.

Royle, J.A. and Walsh, M. (1993) *Watson's Medical–Surgical Nursing and Related Physiology*, 4th edn. London: Baillière-Tindall.

Russell, J.G.B. (1982) The rationale of primitive delivery positions. *British Journal of Obstetrics and Gynaecology*, 89, 712–15.

Russell, K. (2008) Watching and waiting: the facilitation of birth at home. In Edwins, J. (ed.) *Community Midwifery Practice*. Oxford: Blackwell Publishing, pp. 25–45.

Shorten, A., Donsante, J. and Shorten, B. (2002) Birth position, accoucheur, and perineal outcomes: informing women about choices for vaginal birth. *Birth* 29, 18–27.

Simkin, P. and Bolding, A. (2004) Update on non-pharmacologic approaches to relieve labour pain and prevent suffering. *Journal of Midwifery and Women's Health*, 49, 489–504.

Simkin, P. and O'Hara, M. (2002) Non-pharmacological methods of pain relief during labour: systematic review of five methods. *American Journal of Obstetrics and Gynaecology*, 186, S131–59.

Simkin, P. and Klaus, P. (2004) *When Survivors Give Birth: Understanding and Healing the Effects of Early Sexual Abuse on Childbearing Women*. Seattle: Classic Day Publishing.

Spiby, H., Henderson, B., Slade, P., Escott, D. and Fraser, R. (1999) Strategies for coping with labour: does antenatal education translate into practice? *Journal of Advanced Nursing*, 29, 388–94.

Sofaer, B. (1992) *Pain: A Handbook for Nurses: A Pyschophysiologic Approach*, 2nd edn. London: Chapman & Hall.

Steen, M. (2007) Wellbeing and beyond. *RCM Midwives*, 10(3), 116–19.

Steen, M. and Calvert, J. (2006) Homeopathy for childbirth: remedies and research. *RCM Midwives*, 9, 438–40.

Steen, M. and Calvert, J. (2007) A follow up study of women's experiences of using self administration homeopathic remedies. *British Journal of Midwifery*, 15, 359–65.

Sutton, J. (2000) Occipito posterior positioning and some ideas about how to change it. *Practising Midwife*, 3(6), 20–2.

Tarkka, M.J., Paunonen, M. and Laippala, P. (2000). Importance of the midwife in the first-time mother's experience of childbirth. *Scandinavian Journal of Caring Science*, 14, 184–90.

Thomas V.N. (1997) *Pain: Its Nature and Management*. London: Baillière-Tindall.

Tiran, D. (2000) *Clinical Aromatherapy for Pregnancy and Childbirth*, 2nd edn. Edinburgh: Churchill Livingstone.

Tiran, D. (2006) Midwives responsibilities when caring for women using complementary therapies during labour. *MIDIRS Midwifery Digest*, 16(1), 77–8.

Tiran, D. (2010) *Reflexology in Pregnancy and Childbirth*. Edinburgh: Churchill Livingstone.

Tiran, D. and Mack, S. (2000) *Complementary Therapies for Pregnancy and Childbirth*, 2nd edn. London: Harcourt Publishers.

Tunstall, M.E. (1961) Obstetric analgesia: the use of a fixed nitrous oxide and oxygen mixture from one cylinder. Preliminary Communication. *The Lancet* 964.

Walsh, D. (2006) Subverting assembly-line birth: childbirth in a free-standing birth centre. *Social Science and Medicine*, 62, 1330–40.

Walsh, D. (2007) *Evidence-Based Care for Normal Labour and Birth: A Guide for Midwives*. London: Routledge.

Watkins, S.S. (2001) Get on the ball: the 'birth ball' that is! *International Journal of Childbirth Education*, 16(4), 17–19.

Windsor, M. and Laska, M. (2002) *The Pilates Pregnancy*. London: Vermilion.

Wockel, A., Schafer, E., Beggel, A. and Abou-Dakn, M (2007) Getting ready for birth: impending fatherhood. *British Journal of Midwifery*, 15, 344–8.

Yates, S. and Anderson, T. (2003) *Shiatsu for Midwives*. London: Books for Midwives.

Chapter 8   **Case studies**

Mary Steen and Kath Jones

Introduction

This chapter focuses on eight women's homebirth and en route experiences.* The experiences demonstrate eight different outcomes in the home setting. The first woman had a normal birth with no complications. The second woman needed to be transferred to a consultant-led unit. The third woman's baby was 'born before arrival' (BBA). The fourth woman gave birth unexpectedly to a Down's syndrome baby. The fifth woman (a grand multigravida) had a homebirth against medical advice. The sixth woman, who had multiple sclerosis (MS) and was in remission, requested a waterbirth at home and gave birth there against medical advice. The seventh woman had an undiagnosed breech birth. Finally, the eighth woman gave birth en route to hospital. The midwifery care and support given to these women is described and discussed, as is how all eight women reflected on their birth experiences. Regardless of the outcome, mode of delivery or setting, they all described their care and birth positively.

> The best way I know to counter the effects of frightening stories is to hear or read empowering one.
>
> (Gaskin, 2008, p. 4)

Case studies

1. Homebirth – no complications

Maggie was a 26-year-old multigravida and this was her second pregnancy. She had a little boy aged two years and gave birth to him in a hospital setting. She found the experience traumatic and she did not feel in control of her birth. She described the delivery room as hostile and restrictive. She wanted to be as active as possible while in labour, but the delivery room made this difficult for her to achieve and she was encouraged to lie on the bed and give birth in the conventional position. She remembers how painful this was, especially in her lower back, and how she wanted to get up and lean forward. She did not want this to happen to her this time round so she opted for a homebirth. The pregnancy was uneventful and she was seen by her midwife approximately seven times, as recommended by the National Institute for Health and Clinical Excellent (NICE) antenatal guidelines. A home visit was undertaken at 36 weeks to discuss her homebirth.

---

* Pseudonyms have been used to protect the women's anonymity.

Maggie's birth story

I was about 11 days overdue by my dates (my dates and the scan date did not agree) and my midwife arranged a home visit to give me an antenatal check and to also undertake a vaginal examination to perform a 'stretch and sweep' of my cervix as there is apparently some evidence that many women will go into labour within the next 48 hours following this. That was yesterday and since then I have had a couple of shows (jelly-like substance with a streak of blood) and some irregular contractions. Then early this morning I woke up in the early hours, about 3.00 a.m., feeling contractions every 20 minutes or so. I tried to go back to sleep but I couldn't, so I got up and had a warm bath (I put a couple of drops of lavender oil in the bath) to help me relax. At about 4.00 a.m. I took a couple of paracetamol and went back to bed for a few hours and rested. My little boy awoke at about 6.30 a.m. (as usual) so I got up with him and gave him some breakfast. I was becoming increasingly aware that my contractions were now every 10 minutes and getting stronger so my husband decided to stay at home and not go to work and await events.

At approximately 9.00 a.m. my contractions were every five to six minutes, getting stronger and lasting longer, about 60 seconds. My husband called my midwife to let her know that I was in early labour and she confirmed that she would be at our home in the next hour. She advised us to stay calm and for me to remain as active as I possibly could be and use different positions in labour. In the meantime my husband helped me to apply the transcutaneous electrical nerve stimulation (TENS) machine (four pads and electrodes attached to my lower back) and I initially put the TENS on a low setting. The TENS therapy helped me to remain focused and cope with the contractions. I also found it helpful to rock my pelvis backwards and forwards and then from side to side while I stood, and sometimes using the birth ball also helped. My husband was really supportive and encouraged me to stay focused. He massaged my shoulders and just under my abdomen where I was feeling pain the most. The heat from his hands was very soothing and I felt safe and secure. My little boy also held my hand and gave me a kiss and cuddle.

At 9.40 a.m., my midwife arrived and checked my blood pressure, pulse and temperature and felt my abdomen and listened to my baby's heart. Everything was fine and I needed to pass urine as I hadn't done so in the last couple of hours and my midwife wanted to test this as well. Emptying my bladder relieved some of the pressure that I was feeling in my pubic area. My midwife then performed a vaginal examination to assess and confirm that I was in established labour. The examination showed that I was about 5 cm dilated, my cervix was thinning and my baby's head was well applied to my cervix, and my waters were still intact, my baby's heart rate was around 146 beats/min. I was happy to continue walking around, leaning forward and using my kitchen worktop counter for support when I felt a contraction starting. I remember my husband putting a CD on. It was one he had put together for me especially with some of my favourite tunes, which helped me to remain relaxed.

By 10.50 a.m., I was experiencing contractions every two minutes; they were very strong and lasted about 60–70 seconds. I decided to change position, walk around and then march on the spot. My mum arrived and offered to take my little boy to the park and then give him some lunch. I was starting to feel all hot and bothered at this stage. I needed a cool drink with some ice that I could suck, which my husband gave me. I can recall my midwife applying a cool wet cloth to my face and around my neck, and this felt wonderful. I then found comfort from kneeling on all fours and rocking my pelvis. I arched my back into the 'angry cat' position, which helped me work through some contractions.

At around 11.30 am, my contractions became very strong and I wanted to use some gas and air. My midwife sorted this out for me. I inhaled the gas and air using a mouthpiece that was attached to the piping and cylinder. I remember inhaling as my contraction started so that I would feel the effect when my contraction was at its strongest. I used the gas and air for every other contraction as I still liked to walk around and use the TENS machine. My midwife intermittently listened to my baby's heart and everything was fine.

About midday, I felt pressure in my bottom and some urges to push; my waters broke and my contractions were really strong and seemed to be coming every minute, then continuously; there weren't any gaps between them. At this stage, I felt panicky and fearful and didn't think I could cope any more. I remember my midwife being very calm and reassuring and telling me that everything was fine and that I was nearly there. I was going through the 'transition period' and my baby would be born very soon. My husband comforted me and gave me a much needed cuddle. I can still hear his voice encouraging me to remain focused and visualise my baby coming through the birth canal, which I did. He helped me to regain some confidence and reminded me to breathe slowly and steadily. I did this and then felt the urge to push my baby out. My midwife checked to see if I was ready to do so and I was. Thinking back, I don't know where I got my energy from, but I was able to bear down and I felt my baby's head moving down. I recall taking one long last breath, concentrating and pushing my baby out into the world. I felt so relieved and overcome with emotion. My baby girl was born at 12.15 p.m. and my husband cut the cord a few couple of minutes later. I remember feeling exhilarated that I was a mum again. Fantastic! I decided to deliver my placenta (afterbirth) without any drugs and my midwife advised me to put my baby to my breast as this apparently stimulates oxytocin, the hormone that naturally helps to deliver your placenta. My placenta was delivered about 12.45 p.m. I had some pain when my womb contracted, which I was told were 'afterpains'. I didn't remember getting them after my first birth but they weren't too bad. I would recommend having a homebirth to women who are fit and well.

Midwife's comments

Maggie and her husband were well prepared for the birth; they had the confidence to have their baby at home. It was Maggie's second baby and she had previously had a normal birth without any complications. Maggie did what comes naturally and gave birth to a lovely baby girl, weighing 8 lbs 2 oz. She remained active for most of her labour, adopting different postures and positions, and used a birth ball to help her cope. Her husband was very supportive and they worked as a team. Maggie was in control of her birth; she remained focused. Her breathing was slow and steady, music helped her to remain calm and she found the TENS machine very helpful. When her contractions were coming every minute and very strong she used Entonox, which helped her cope. When she was going through the transition period (end of the first stage of labour) she did panic a little and felt she could not take any more. This is quite normal, but her husband and I gave her extra support and encouraged her to stay focused, and she worked with her body's natural instincts, found inner strength and had a normal birth. She gently lifted her baby to her breast and her baby suckled. She had a physiological third stage (no drugs) and her placenta and membranes were delivered approximately 26 minutes after the birth. Her labour was about nine hours from start to finish, and this is normal for a second-time mum. It was a privilege to be at the birth.

2. Homebirth – transfer to a consultant-led unit

At 8.00 a.m., a community midwife was contacted and informed by the community team leader that a 32-year-old primigravida woman (Ann) who was low risk and booked for homebirth had contacted the delivery suite to inform them that she might be in labour. She was term plus three days and her contractions were every five minutes, but they were not very strong or, as Ann described it, 'nothing to write home about', and her waters were still intact. The midwife arrived at Ann's home at 8.30 a.m., and found her to be coping well and indeed in established labour.

Ann's birth story

I was a couple of days overdue and had been niggling for the last few days but I was now becoming aware that these niggles were becoming stronger and more regular. I had a warm bath and settled for the night. I awoke at about 4.00 a.m., and got up for the toilet and noticed a jelly-like pink-stained discharge which I assumed was a show. I felt some mild contractions and decided to take two paracetamol tablets and go back to bed. I tossed and turned for while but managed to doze off about 5.00 a.m. I reawoke at about 6.30 a.m., and felt that my contractions were becoming more regular. My partner got up to make a cup of tea and timed my contractions as being every 8–10 minutes. I decided to have another warm bath, which was soothing and relaxing. By 7.30 a.m. my contractions, although of similar intensity, were lasting longer and I remained active and walked around the living room. My partner massaged my back and put a meditation CD on. By 8.00 a.m., my contractions were every five minutes, and lasting a good minute, but I was coping well. At this stage I decided to contact the delivery suite as instructed to arrange for a midwife to come to my home.

At about 8.30 a.m., a community midwife arrived at my home. I hadn't met her before but she introduced herself and greeted me warmly. She asked me to tell her in my own words what the contractions felt like and she palpated the contractions. She took some observations and listened to my baby's heart beat. I needed help to apply the TENS machine as my partner wasn't sure where to place the pads. The midwife sorted this out and I started to use it on a low setting. We had a cup of tea and I asked to be examined; I wanted to know if I was in labour. The midwife said I was and she would examine me to see how I was progressing. I was 5 cm dilated and my cervix was thinning out nicely; my baby's head was engaged but still had some way to descend.

For the next couple of hours I remained active, marching on the spot and gently rocking my pelvis. Everything seemed to be going fine and the midwife contacted the delivery suite to say she was staying with me. About 2.00 p.m. I was feeling tired and decided to have a lie down but could not get comfortable, so I had another warm bath, which did help. An hour or so later the contractions were getting stronger and I needed something stronger than the TENS machine. The midwife arranged for the gas and air to be delivered. At about 4.00 p.m. I started using the gas and air and increased the intensity setting on the TENS machine. At 6.00 p.m. I was starting to feel panicky and was feeling urges to push. The midwife re-examined me and found that I was 8 cm dilated and my cervix was continuing to thin out. My partner prepared a small fruit salad for me, which was lovely – I felt energised! I remember catnapping between the contractions, another cylinder of gas and air arriving and being re-examined about 8.00 p.m. I was still 8 cm dilated, which disappointed me, but my waters broke at this point. I was getting tired but still coping well. A small fibroid had been detected on ultrasound during my pregnancy and my midwife was wondering whether it had grown and was possibly obstructing the descent of my baby through the birth canal. She contacted the hospital to ask another midwife to attend.

Two midwives arrived as they had just come on duty and were members of the homebirth team. The midwife who had been with me all day handed over care. I was re-examined an hour later but was still 8 cm dilated and had not progressed. At this stage it was decided that I should be transferred to the delivery suite. On arrival an obstetrician came to see me and examined me: still no progress, but my baby was fine. I remember the obstetrician saying that we would watch and wait. I was struggling to cope now and an epidural was sited. A drip to help establish my contractions again was also sited. At about 10.30 p.m., the obstetrician discussed the need to intervene and told me that my temperature was high. Half an hour or so later, I was in theatre having a caesarean section. My partner was with me throughout. I gave birth to a lovely little boy. I wasn't too disappointed that I had a caesarean and not a homebirth as planned and I would describe my baby's birth as a positive experience. I had laboured at home and felt safe, in control and well supported during that time. Equally, I felt safe and well cared for in the delivery suite. Everyone involved in my care explained and discussed what was happening and I was happy to be transferred when the need arose.

Midwife's comments

Ann and her partner coped very well; Ann's labour was progressing well but a problem became apparent when she was 8 cm dilated. Her baby's head was more than 2 cm above the ischial spines and not descending. Interestingly, her own mother had failed to progress and had a caesarean when giving birth to Ann 32 years previously. The fibroid was a cause for concern and she was getting tired. She was happy to be transferred to the delivery suite and understood why a caesarean section was indicated. She felt that she had laboured and everyone concerned supported her in her choice to have a planned homebirth but the appropriate actions were taken when intervention became necessary. She describes her birth experience as a positive one.

3. Homebirth – born before arrival (BBA)

Julie was a 22-year-old multigravida and had a 24-hour labour with her first baby. She was fit and well during this second pregnancy and booked for a hospital birth. She was term plus four days and had a precipitate delivery at home. Her partner and friend were with her when she gave birth on her bathroom floor. Emergency services and a community midwife were on their way but Julie delivered her baby girl very quickly.

Julie's birth story

During the night I had felt irregular contractions, but nothing to write home about. When I awoke about 7.30 a.m. I had backache and mild pain. I carried on as usual and took my little boy to nursery. I was planning on going shopping with my friend Michelle but felt a little unwell and so we decided to stay at my home for a coffee and a chat. Just as well, as all of a sudden I started to feel very strong contractions and felt sick. It was about 11.30 a.m. and I phoned my partner John to come home from work as I was sure I was in labour. In the meantime, I decided to have a bath and a couple of paracetamols to ease the pain. Michelle helped me into the bath and the pains seemed to ease off a bit. John arrived home and was making a cup of tea when I started to feel the urge to push.

John helped me out of the bath and I had another strong contraction. I was starting to panic and John contacted the delivery suite for advice. I vaguely remember John telling me that an ambulance and a midwife were on their way. I remember thinking please get here quickly my baby is on her way. The urge to push was getting stronger and I was getting very distressed. Michelle came running in and helped me to get onto the bathroom floor. Everything happened so fast, it was surreal; I was pushing my baby's head out and I remember thinking this cannot be happening, I have not been in labour that long. With another strong contraction, my baby girl was born. John wrapped her in a towel and we waited for help to arrive.

About 10 minutes later, a paramedic arrived and checked to see if my baby and I were all right. It was about another 15 minutes or so when the midwife arrived. She reassured me and quickly delivered my placenta. My blood loss was okay, but I needed some stitches, which the midwife sorted out. I was shaking and shivering, obviously suffering from shock. I expected to be in labour for hours as I had been with my first baby. The midwife stayed with me for a while and gave my baby a warm feed and checked her over. We were both fine and I was happy that I didn't have to go into hospital and could stay at home.

Midwife's comments

Julie had a precipitate delivery and went on to give birth at home with no midwife in attendance. The emergency services arrived 10 minutes after she had given birth and the midwife, who had to drive from the other side of the city to get to Julie's home, arrived about 15 minutes later. She was on the bathroom floor and in a state of shock. Her placenta was delivered physiologically. Her observations and blood loss were normal and her uterus was well contracted. Vaginal examination revealed that she had sustained a second-degree tear. I gave a local anaesthetic to numb the perineal region and sutured the second-degree tear and then helped her into the bath. Julie had a warm drink and something light to eat. Her baby girl was alert and warm. After checking her baby's observations, I proceeded to give her a warm feed. I stayed approximately two hours, completed the necessary paperwork and then went to the delivery suite to notify the birth and to dispose of the placenta and clinical waste. I returned at 5.00 p.m. to check that all was well, left contact numbers and arranged a visit for the next day.

4. Homebirth – Down's syndrome baby

Lucy was a 35-year-old multigravida. She had had two normal births in hospital and had decided at the booking interview to have a homebirth. She was well supported by her husband and family. She went into spontaneous labour at term plus two days and was attended at home by two midwives whom she had not previously met. She laboured in her bedroom and was mobile throughout. She used Entonox as pain relief. She went on to all fours to give birth and after 10 minutes of active pushing gave birth to a baby girl.

Lucy's story

I knew something was wrong straight away! I had declined the triple test during my pregnancy as I would not have considered having an amniocentesis or termination if there had been something wrong. The two midwives did not convey their concerns to me. I got into bed with my husband Ray at my side. The two midwives left us alone and went to make some tea. On their return one of the midwives asked me what I thought of my daughter. I responded, 'Do you think she has Down's syndrome?' The midwife replied that she thought she did. I was worried that she would not be able to breast-feed, but one of the midwives helped me to latch her on and she fed well for about 30 minutes. I was warned that my baby might have to go into hospital. The midwife explained to me that although the baby would need to see a paediatrician, she had good Apgar scores and had fed well so there was no immediate rush. The midwives stayed for a couple of hours after birth to monitor the baby and arranged for one of them to visit early the next day. My husband and I were made aware that if there were any problems with the baby's colour, feeding or breathing we should phone the emergency services (999). The labour ward was informed of the birth. The following day the consultant paediatrician was contacted and an appointment to see him the next day was arranged. My husband and I were in shock, and having to come to terms with the fact that our baby girl had Down's syndrome was difficult, but being at home in our own familiar surroundings with our other children helped.

Midwife's comments

Lucy and her husband talked of the shock of having a baby with Down's syndrome but also how being at home and being able to see this for themselves made what could have been a tragedy into a positive birth experience. The children were told of the baby's condition and bonded well with her immediately.

At the next homebirth risk assessment meeting, which is held monthly at the maternity unit, this case study was discussed in great depth. Many midwives and an obstetrician expressed concern that this baby was not immediately transferred into hospital as there was great risk of heart anomalies and potential feeding problems. The physical risks seemed to outweigh emotional, social and environmental risks. The decision to keep her at home was made on the basis that the baby appeared well and had good Apgar scores and that vital signs were within normal range. Within an hour of giving birth the baby had a good breast-feed and, apart from the possibility of Down's syndrome, was showing no signs of having any other problems. Keeping the baby with the family meant that, although they were aware of difficult times ahead, they were able to enjoy the birth experience as a family.

5. Homebirth – against medical advice

Helen was a 38-year-old woman who was pregnant for the seventh time. She had an obstetric history of six normal uncomplicated pregnancies resulting in normal births. However, both her third and fourth children had suffered apnoea attacks and dusky episodes in the first few hours after birth. These subsided, and her two children have grown and developed normally and are healthy. Helen's fifth and sixth children did not experience any such episodes. Helen had expressed a desire to give birth at home to the fifth and sixth children, but her husband had been reluctant in case there were any complications. At the booking interview Helen stated that this was to be her last baby and that she would like a homebirth. Her husband was very supportive.

Helen was advised that, because she was a 'grand multipara', there were risks associated with homebirth and that homebirth policy advised against homebirth after four deliveries. Despite being made aware of the risks, Helen was determined to go ahead. The same community midwife had attended her during all her previous pregnancies and she felt confident that this midwife had the skills and ability to care for her. She stressed that if at any time her labour deviated from normal she would agree to hospital admission.

Helen's birth story

I live with my family in a farmhouse which is in the process of being renovated and which is accessed via a single-track mountain road. The farmhouse is not easily accessible by car, but owning a Land Rover helps. I was aware of some risks if I had a homebirth but I was also aware of the benefits. My community midwife discussed the risks with me and carried out a full risk assessment supported by a supervisor of midwives. The problem of access was addressed. An ambulance could access the property and my husband would come to the top of the road to pick up the midwives. I had a land line and mobile phone and a map was provided for midwives on call. My eldest child was 15 years old and would be able to look after the other children. My parents also lived nearby and were willing to help.

I was due in early autumn so the weather should not prove to be a problem. In preparation, copies of the risk assessment were given to all the on-call midwives. My pregnancy progressed normally and at 28 weeks a blood sample to measure my haemoglobin level was fine (12.7 g/dl). My baby was very active with good fetal movements and growth was reassuring. My baby was head down from around 34 weeks. I was offered a membrane sweep at term and then a week later.

Following the second membrane sweep I went into labour about eight hours later. Luckily, my community midwife was on call and when she arrived at my home it was clearly evident that I was in established labour.

All my observations were within normal limits and I was contracting for one minute every five. I did not need any pain relief as I was coping well in an upright position and rocking my pelvis during the contractions. The second midwife arrived at the top of the track and my husband left to fetch her. During the 10 minutes he was away, I suddenly had urges to push and quickly delivered our baby boy. By the time my husband arrived back, I was in bed and breast-feeding. My blood loss was minimal and my midwife said my baby had good Apgar scores. My husband said he wasn't too disappointed at not being there as he felt it was more important that I had had the birth I wanted. Our other children came into the bedroom straight away to see their new brother, which was wonderful!

I had always felt that I had missed out somehow by having hospital births. A few of my friends had expressed to me how positive homebirths were and I wanted the experience. I was delighted to have been supported by my community midwife and the local maternity services. My homebirth was absolutely wonderful, thank you.

Midwife's comments

This case study highlights that as long as there a rigorous risk assessment is undertaken and there is good communication between the midwife and the woman to deal with any physical, emotional, social or environmental problems, women can be supported in their choice of a homebirth and have a positive experience.

The physical risks were addressed:

- *Unstable lie.* Helen agreed that in the case of malposition or malpresentation of the baby she would be transferred to hospital.
- *Postpartum haemorrhage (PPH).* Helen agreed to active management of the third stage. Two ampoules of Syntometrine and one of ergometrine were available. She had successfully breast-fed all her children and she always fed as soon as possible after birth following skin-to-skin contact.

6. Homebirth – waterbirth

Mandy, a 28-year-old primigravida who was diagnosed with multiple sclerosis at the age of 24 had a waterbirth in her own familiar home surroundings. She had no problems with her pregnancy and had antenatal appointments with her midwife approximately 10 times as recommended by the antenatal NICE guidelines and with a consultant obstetrician at 20 weeks gestation. Owing to her medical condition she was categorised as high risk and the risks and benefits of a homebirth were discussed with her. She used hydrotherapy frequently to ease pain she sometimes felt in her limbs and a waterbirth was in her opinion her best option. A waterbirth in the consultant-led unit was discussed but she was adamant that she wanted to be in her own home. A risk assessment was completed and her community midwife had support from her supervisor of midwives. At her 36-week antenatal appointment, the midwife discussed Mandy's birth plan and how she was planning to manage her labour. She had set her heart on having a waterbirth in her own home.

Mandy's birth story

During my pregnancy I was labelled high risk as I suffer from multiple sclerosis. I do not consider myself to be high risk. I am in remission and feel fit and well. Yes, I struggle with walking and sometimes have to use a stick but I didn't see any reason why I couldn't have a waterbirth at home as I use hydrotherapy frequently to ease my joint pains. A waterbirth in hospital was offered but after all the appointments and treatments I have received over the last few years I have a fear of going anywhere near a hospital. I considered that having my baby in water at home was less risky for me than giving birth in hospital and that I would be able to cope better.

When I was four days past my expected date of delivery I felt some lower backache and experienced irregular contractions. I had a show the day before. I began to feel my contractions becoming more regular and getting uncomfortable. I woke up about 7.00 a.m. feeling my abdomen tightening and then I became aware that I was having some regular contractions. I used some breathing techniques I had been shown at an antenatal class and I remained active and adopted different positions to help me cope. I used a birth ball at home until my contractions were five minutes apart and lasting a good minute. I decide to ring my midwife as I was feeling a little anxious, unsure and thought I needed to use the birth pool to help me relax, remain focused and stay calm. The midwife informed me that she was on her way and told me to get my partner to help me get the pool ready.

At 11.35 a.m., my midwife arrived and greeted me warmly. She palpated my abdomen and timed my contractions, she listened to my baby's heart rate and, with my permission, performed a vaginal examination. She confirmed that I was in established labour and progressing well. She informed me that I was approximately 5 cm dilated and my cervix was about 50 per cent effaced. My forewaters were starting to form and my baby's head was descending. At 12.10 p.m. I got into the birth pool and it felt wonderful! I was able to gently move around and change my position as I had space and flexibility to do so. The warm water eased my backache and the tight cramp-like pains I was experiencing and I felt calmer and started to relax my body. I focused on my labour positively and knew I had the ability to give birth naturally in my safe home environment. I found kneeling in the water and gently rocking my pelvis backwards and forwards and then from side to side very helpful. My partner was really supportive and encouraged me to work with my body. He embraced me and whispered encouraging words in my ear, which made me feel secure and safe.

Periodically, I was aware that the midwife was listening to my baby's heart rate and that everything was fine. At 3.20 p.m. my contractions were coming every one to two minutes and were very strong. At this point I had a little panic attack and felt some doubt about my ability to cope. I was reassured by my midwife and my partner that I was doing fantastically well and that my baby would be born soon. I managed to get focused again and at 3.40 p.m. I felt the urge to bear down and push.

At 3.52 p.m., I felt my baby's head being born and a couple of minutes later I pushed my baby out into the warm water. The midwife gently lifted my baby up towards me and we both remain submerged in the water and enjoyed our first few moments together. I decided to get out of the pool and I had a physiological third stage (no drugs) and put my baby to my breast to help this process. At 4.20 p.m. my afterbirth was delivered and I did not need any stitches. I felt wonderful and would recommend a waterbirth to women who want to give birth naturally.

Midwife's comments

Hydrotherapy has been used for many years to alleviate aches and pains and using a birthing pool during labour is an excellent way for some women to achieve pain relief. Mandy was used to hydrotherapy and had confidence in its ability to ease pain and discomfort. In addition, the warm water helped her to remain calm and relaxed. She was able to cope with her labour pains and was able to move around and adopt different positions and the water helped her be buoyant. Her partner was able to hold her and make her feel safe and secure. Mandy and her partner were very focused and worked as a pair; this helped her progress in labour quickly and her labour was approximately nine hours and 20 minutes from start to finish. Mandy's birth was wonderful to observe and I would recommend that women should think about using a birthing pool during childbirth as an option in both the home and hospital setting.

7. Homebirth – undiagnosed breech birth

Lowri was a 33-year-old woman expecting her third baby. Her two previous pregnancies had been normal. Her second child was BBA at home, as she had been sent home from hospital after being told she was not in labour. She decided that this time she would have a planned homebirth and be prepared. Her pregnancy was uneventful and she went into spontaneous labour at term plus five days.

Palpation revealed a cephalic presentation. A vaginal examination showed that Lowri was 4 cm dilated with a high presentation and bulging membranes; the baby's position was indeterminate.

Lowri laboured well without any pain relief and was relaxed throughout. Her children were in bed and her husband Neil was with her. She announced that she had urges to push and sat forward on the sofa. At this point the midwife noted bulging membranes and a visible plug of meconium. Lowri delivered a baby girl in the frank breech presentation. The baby's Apgar score was 9 at both one minute and five minutes. She breast-fed well soon after birth.

I decided to have a homebirth more for my husband than for me. He was traumatised by the birth of our second son, as he had delivered him at home under instructions from ambulance control. I was looked after by my community midwife, who had cared for me in the last pregnancy, and she agreed to be on call for the birth as she knew how anxious we were not to be on our own again.

When I was examined I told her I thought I could feel a foot under my ribs. She felt it too and guided my hand around the outline. When I needed to push she told me 'I think the bottom is coming first'. I asked her if that was OK and she reassured me that it was fine.

My waters broke and Sian was delivered in two pushes. It felt no different to giving birth head first. We were all delighted and she fed straight away. This was an added bonus as I had not been able to feed my sons. Neil was very calm throughout and, because the midwives did not convey any anxiety, we did not realise that there could have been problems with a breech birth. It was a very special experience which helped to wipe out the previous trauma.

Following this birth, I discussed the case with my supervisor of midwives and completed a personal reflection. On reflection, I realised that I had been misguided by feeling the baby's feet in the upper part of the uterus when in fact the baby was in a frank breech position. Nor was I alerted when I felt bulging membranes and was unable to determine the baby's position. Fortunately, I was aware that Lowri had delivered two 4-kg babies previously and was not concerned that delivery would be a problem. The birth was so quick there was not a great deal of time to ponder. She lived 30 minutes from the maternity unit so transfer would not be possible at full dilation.

Lowri was sitting on the edge of the sofa so this was an ideal position for birth. I had not delivered a breech baby at home before but I had recently attended an emergency skills drill study day and practised delivering a baby in the frank breech position. This helped me to clearly remember 'hands off the breech' and remain calm. I patiently 'watched and waited' for the baby's buttocks to descend through the birth canal. Lowri delivered her baby with minimal assistance from me; I only needed to gently support her baby's head as it was born (see Chapter 5).

This case was discussed at the homebirth risk meeting. I was able to share my experience and identify where I had misinterpreted the palpation and vaginal examination. We discussed transfer to hospital if the diagnosis of breech presentation had been made earlier. Fortunately for Lowri she was too late. She admitted that she would not have agreed to go to hospital and a possible Caesarean Section, so both parents and midwives were spared the anxiety of dealing with that situation. It also reaffirmed to me that skills learned in breech delivery can be successfully implemented in practice.

8. Homebirth – birth en route

Kim was a 21-year-old multigravida who had had two previous normal births with minimal intervention. She was fit and well during this third pregnancy and booked for a hospital birth. She was 38 weeks and 2 days gestation when she spontaneously went into labour at home. She called her midwife, who was undertaking an antenatal clinic at her local health centre, to inform her that she was in early labour; her contractions were every 8–10 minutes, lasting about one minute. The midwife arranged to do a home visit after her clinic and discussed being active during labour and advised using the birth ball. A trusting relationship had developed between the woman and midwife during the previous pregnancies and birth. This case study is an excellent example of how continuity of care and carer is beneficial and appreciated.

Kim's birth story

Early in the morning about 5.30 a.m., I felt irregular contractions that were not painful. I took a couple of paracetamol and dozed off for another hour or so. When I woke up again, it was about 7.00 a.m. and the irregular contractions were becoming regular, every 10–15 minutes. My partner went to work at 7.30 a.m. and I got my two children their breakfast. I rang my mother to let her know that I thought I was in early labour and asked if she could come around to help look after her grandchildren and support me. My mother arrived about 8.45 a.m. and decided that she would take my elder child, Emma, to school and my younger, Thomas, to the park. This would give me some free time to have a relaxing bath. About midday, my contractions were becoming more frequent, about every 10 minutes, but were not very painful. My mother returned with Thomas and I prepared a light lunch (sandwiches and some fruit).

It was about 1 p.m. when I telephoned my midwife at the local health centre. I knew she would be there as she had an antenatal clinic from 1 to 3.30 pm on that day. She arranged to visit me at home after the clinic and advised that I should remain as active as possible, use my birth ball and ring her back if I thought I was cracking on. My midwife had cared for me during my two previous pregnancies and was with me when I gave birth to my first baby (Emma) when I was only 15. She was on leave when I had my second baby (Thomas) when I was aged 19 and, even though I received good care, I missed her. I trusted my midwife and felt safe and cared for; I was pleased she was on duty.

I kept myself busy and telephoned my partner to say that I was in labour and my midwife was going to call about 4 p.m. so he didn't have to rush home – he could finish his shift! About 3.00 p.m., I had a catnap and my mother went to pick Emma up from school and then I watched television with my children. At 4 p.m., my midwife arrived; my contractions were becoming stronger and more frequent, approximately every three to five minutes, lasting a good minute. My midwife confirmed that I was in labour and about 5–6 cm dilated. I needed to go into hospital. My hospital bag was ready and I telephoned my partner to meet me at the hospital. My contractions were now every two to five minutes and very strong; I was finding it difficult to cope. My midwife telephoned for an ambulance, which arrived about 4.30 p.m., and I was transferred to the maternity unit. I remember using gas and air in the ambulance and my midwife massaging my lower back. I also remember a paramedic saying that the traffic was busy and the blue light was flashing and I could hear the siren. I was feeling the urge to push with each contraction now and I was becoming anxious. My midwife reminded me to breathe slowly and not to panic; I knew I was in safe hands. She asked the ambulance driver to pull over into the lay-by. I gave birth in the ambulance to a lovely baby girl. Apparently, it is believed that she will be lucky in life as she was born in her bag of water (which I later learned is described as *en caul*). I remember my midwife giving me an injection to help deliver my placenta and also saying we could turn around and go back home as everything was fine but I wanted to go into hospital as I needed a well-earned rest!

Midwife's comments

I had cared for Kim during her two previous pregnancies and supported her in labour with her first baby when she was a teenager. Therefore, I had built up a trusting relationship with her and her family. She would have been an ideal candidate for a homebirth but her choice was to have a hospital birth and stay over night. Kim was 38+2 days gestation and I had only just seen her two days previously at an antenatal clinic appointment. She was healthy and had no problems during her pregnancy. I had just arrived at the health centre to commence an antenatal clinic when I got a telephone call from Kim. She was in early labour and I arranged to visit her at home after I had finished the clinic. I advised her that, in the meantime, she should ring me if she had any concerns; I discussed remaining active and using the birth ball. I knew her mother was there to help with Emma and Thomas and it was likely that she would progress steadily and go into established labour. At 4 p.m. I arrived at

Kim's home and found that she had progressed and was in established labour. Her contractions were every three to five minutes and were strong and lasting 60–70 seconds. She was coping very well and walking around. Her observations were satisfactory and on vaginal examination her cervix was almost effaced and 5–6 cm dilated. The baby's head was well applied and Kim's waters were intact. The fetal heart was regular at 140–146 beats/min. I called for the ambulance, which arrived at approximately 4.30 p.m. Kim had her overnight bag ready and I accompanied her in the ambulance to the maternity unit. I was aware that traffic was busy and that the ambulance driver had switched on the emergency blue light and siren to try and get through the traffic.

Kim was feeling the urge to bear down and push, I knew birth was imminent and asked the ambulance driver to pull over into a lay-by. Kim gave birth at 5.02 p.m. to a live baby girl in the amniotic sac of water, which spontaneously ruptured as her baby was born and took her first breath. The baby's Apgar scores were good: 8 at one minute and 9 at five minutes. The placenta was delivered at 5.08 p.m. following active management. We arrived at the maternity unit at 5.20 p.m. Both Kim and the baby (Angela) were doing fine. Kim stayed overnight and returned home the next day and continued to have midwifery care.

Conclusions

This chapter has given an insight into eight women's recent homebirth experiences. The case studies described and discussed clearly demonstrate different issues that woman and midwives can experience in the home setting. The first case study was straightforward and the woman had a normal birth with no complications.

This should inspire women to believe in their own ability to give birth without fear and the need for interventions. In contrast, the second case study was not straightforward and the woman needed to be transferred into a consultant-led unit. However, for most of her labour she was at home in her own familiar surroundings with the support of her partner and a midwife. When a problem was identified the necessary actions were taken and everyone concerned with her care played their part to enable her to experience a positive birth.

The third case study relates to a woman who had booked for a hospital birth but whose baby was 'born before arrival' (BBA) at home. She gave birth with no midwife in attendance. However, emergency and midwifery services were notified and were on their way. She was well supported when the emergency services and midwife arrived and remained at home. The fourth case study involves a woman who gave birth unexpectedly to a Down's syndrome baby.

This woman and her partner were fully supported in their decision to remain at home on the basis that their baby girl's vital signs were satisfactory and she had breast-fed well. This decision meant that, although they were aware of difficult times ahead, they were still able to enjoy the birth experience as a family.

The fifth case study describes and discusses a woman's (grand multigravida) homebirth experience against medical advice. This case study gives an insight into how a woman requesting a homebirth against medical advice can be supported. A risk assessment was undertaken to address physical, emotional, social or environmental issues and ensure that resources and systems were in place as and/or when required. Good communication and a trusting relationship between the woman, her partner and midwife promoted a positive birth experience.

Similarly, the sixth case study involves a woman also giving birth against medical advice. She had multiple sclerosis but was in remission and her request to have a waterbirth at home was supported by maternity services. This a good example of how individual women's needs can be addressed to support them in their birth choices.

The seventh case study describes and discusses a woman who had an undiagnosed breech birth at home. It is a good example of how a breech presentation might be missed on abdominal palpation and when performing a vaginal examination. However, it demonstrates that midwives can facilitate a breech birth in the home setting with confidence and with emergency skills education and training.

Finally, the eighth case study is about a woman who gave birth en route to hospital (in the ambulance). It demonstrates how a trusting relationship with a midwife and continuity of care can positively help a woman to feel safe and supported. This woman could have returned home following the birth in the ambulance but her decision to continue and be admitted to hospital was respected. According to Kizinger (2002, p. 8), 'a good birth is one which the woman looks back on, whatever happened, with satisfaction and fulfilment' and 'Everything that happens during a birth influences the way in which a woman perceives herself afterwards. It can affect the relationship between her and the baby and between both parents and their baby, for years after the actual birth'.

The midwifery care and support given to all these women demonstrates that maternity services and midwives can support women to have a planned or unplanned birth. All eight women reflected on their birth experiences positively even if things did not go as they planned and regardless of the mode of delivery or place of birth. These case studies are good examples of how experienced midwives dealt with different issues that happened when supporting women to have a planned or unplanned homebirth. They had the confidence, skills and resources available to support them in their decision-making and provision of midwifery care in the home setting.

References

Gaskin, I.M. (2008) *Ina May's Guide to Childbirth*. London: Vermilion.
Kitzinger, S. (2002) *Birth Your Way: Choosing Birth at Home or in a Birth Centre*. London: Dorling Kindersley.

Summary

There will always an element of uncertainty around giving birth at home, but being in a hospital setting does not prevent uncertainty either. Absolute safety can not be guaranteed in any birth environment. However, good preparation and planning will help to minimise the risks associated with birth. Education and training regarding both the benefits and risks associated with homebirth are essential and should include how to deal with any issues if and when they arise. Providing a homebirth service and the education and training needs can be problematic for some maternity services in this present climate with on-going financial constraints, staffing issues and limited resources. Some maternity services have introduced homebirth teams and others have given independent midwives contracts to provide local services to address these issues and to support women in their choice to have a homebirth. Providing a homebirth service clearly has many benefits for women; it also gives midwives opportunities to encourage normal birth and support women in their own home. The case studies in the final chapter provide a realistic insight into possible outcomes when a homebirth is planned or unplanned, but what is clearly demonstrated is that all the women reported a positive birth experience, and felt safe and supported, and that is ultimately the aim when caring for women during childbirth.

> All pregnant women deserve the best possible care and advice founded on the best available evidence of effectiveness applied with understanding, empathy and a philosophy of respect for the process of normal pregnancy and birth.
>
> (Hofmeyr *et al.*, 2008, p. XIII)

No doubt there will be different views with regards to providing a homebirth service and the homebirth debate will continue. However, it is midwives who attend homebirths and support women and their families. Midwives need to be 'with woman', and this includes caring and supporting her in her own home and supporting the choice of homebirth as a genuine option.

Reference

Hofmeyr, G.J., Neilson, J.P., Alfirevic Z., Crowther C.A., Gulmezoglu, Hodnett E.D., Gyte G.M.L. and Duley L. (2008) Preface. In *A Cochrane Pocket Book: Pregnancy and Childbirth*. Chichester: John Wiley & Sons.

Index

abdominal palpitations 136, 138, 139

abnormal labour, emergencies and 161–92; adult airway check 184; adult breathing check 184; adult circulation check 184; adult life support, algorithm for 185; baby, emergency resuscitation for 187–92; bimanual compression 183; birth en route 167; born before arrival (BBA) 167, 169; breech presentation 174; cardiac compressions on newborn 191; cardiopulmonary resuscitation (CPR) 186–8; care of mother and baby in emergency 169–83; causes of postpartum haemorrhage (PPH) 181–82; cord compression, prevention of 178; cord prolapse 176–9; delivering baby in breech position 174–6; delivering baby in breech position, guidance for 175–6; diagnosis of postpartum haemorrhage (PPH) 180; emergency resuscitation 183–91; emergency skills drills, importance of 162; fundal massage 183; intervention for postpartum haemorrhage (PPH) 182–3; malpositions and malpresentations 163–5; management of cord prolapse 178–9; mother, emergency resuscitation for 183–7; newborn airway check 188; newborn breathing check 188; newborn circulation check 189–91; newborn life support, algorithm for 191; obstetric emergencies 162; occipitoposterior (OP) position 163–3; postpartum haemorrhage (PPH) 179–83; presenting breech fetus, possible positions 173–4; primary postpartum haemorrhage (PPH) 180–83; resuscitation equipment, availability of 185; Safer Births UK programme 162–3; SBAR (situation, background, assessment, recommendations) 'transfer in' form 167–9; SBAR (situation, background, assessment, recommendations) 'transfer in' form, example of 168; shoulder dystocia 169–73; stimulation of newborn 188–90; stimulation of newborn, basic guidance 189; transfer to consultant-led unit 165–9; undiagnosed breech 173–9

access to homebirths, barriers to 66

Ackermann-Liebrich, U. *et al*. 48

aconite 219

active birth, promotion of 208

activity, benefits of being active 206–7

acupressure 215–16

acupuncture 216–17

adults: airway check 184; breathing check 184; circulation check 184; life support, algorithm for 185

advice provision, art and skill of 22–3

aerobic exercise during pregnancy 206–7

Agnodice 3.

Aikins Murphy, P. and Feinland, J.B. 148

Albers, L.L. 97, 138, 208

Albers, L.L. *et al*. 138, 143, 148

Albrechtsen, S. *et al*. 174

Alehagen, S. *et al*. 91

alternative therapies for pain management 204–25

ambulance service, emergency availability of 38

American College of Obstericians and Gynaecologists 87

American Journal of Obsterics and Gynaecology 87–8

American Medical Association (AMA) 87

amniotomy 136, 140

analgesia 224–5

anatomical atlases, pregnant women as models in 5

ancient Egyptian practices 2

ancient Greek practices 3

Anderson, J.M. and Etches, D. 181

Andrews, A. 21

antenatal care, beginnings of 7